HOW I OVERCAME FIBROMYALGIA
By Edmund S. Figure

Published by Autumn Venture Incorporated,
Macomb, Michigan 48042

Editor: Eileen M. Sandlin

I0429305

First edition January 2012

HOW I OVERCAME FIBROMYALGIA

Contents

GLOSSARY

ABOUT THE AUTHOR

DEDICATION

To my father, who taught me not to accept things the way they are, but rather to strive for something better. To my mother for teaching me how to be patient with people. To my sister for those hours listening on the phone when I was in pain. To my loving wife for always being there for me and helping me through the most difficult time of my life. To my daughter for showing me her youthful enthusiasm for life.

To Dr. John Kowalezyk, Dr. Richard Cicala, Dr. Elizabeth Becker, Dr. Steven Hartz, and Certified Massage Therapist Connie Moore. Without each of you and all of your knowledge, dedication, commitment, and patience I never would have recovered from fibromyalgia.

May God bless all of you!

PREFACE

My father once told me a story about a man who took his car to a mechanic because it wasn't running quite right. He explained that the car idled roughly and sputtered when he stepped on the gas. The mechanic started the car, listened, then took a screw driver and turned a screw on the carburetor. The engine purred and the problem was solved.

"That will be $250" said the mechanic.

"What!" Exclaimed the customer. "$250 for a screwdriver! That's crazy!"

The mechanic calmly looked at the customer.

"The $250 isn't for the screwdriver it is for knowing what to do with it."

I share the story because the analogy is similar to the explanation of fibromyalgia that you will learn about in this book. I'm not going to cure your condition here nor am I going to teach you how to cure yourself.

No for the "princely sum" of this book I am going to share with you how my fibromyalgia developed, what didn't work when I tried to fix it, and then finally how I overcame it.

But even better than that I'm going to help you out with your situation. I'm going to list the specialized doctors in the United States, Canada, and United Kingdom who may be able to help you. In effect that is the "screwdriver" that I am offering you in these pages.

The cost to you for this information is minimal. It is only the cost of this book plus one appointment with a specialist which is often a free initial consultation! Think for a moment. Even this could potentially save you years of anguish looking for a cure. I spent years looking myself—had I had access to this information back then I could have saved decades of pain.

I will also tell you how to do a couple of simple tests to decide for yourself if you can be helped just like I was. This will give you a hint to determine if you can be helped just like I was.

Now suppose none of this helps you out. For a small sum you have eliminated one possible source of your problem. Then you can look elsewhere for a solution. Knowledge can only help you in your position so more knowledge is "win-win" for you.

My fibromyalgia crept up on me over decades culminating in an event that almost destroyed my life. It came in like a thief in the night—I never knew what hit me until it was too late.

What followed was a long struggle through the medical system that left me without an answer but in great pain. Then I got lucky and found the right resource that led me on path to recovery. This recovery was slow and methodical but it worked.

I can only imagine how difficult it must be to take advice from someone you have never met. I have personally talked to many people and advised them this course of action. I've only been able to persuade about half to give it a try. Being a skeptic can be a good thing but don't let it keep you from resolving your health issue.

Of those I talked to who didn't try all are still suffering to this day. Those who followed my advice and were checked out by a specialist all obtained relief. I think that speaks for itself.

On the other hand I understand desperation. I've been there and I know what it is like to be in such immense pain that nothing else matters in your life. When I put down the first words to this book my goal was simple: If I could help just one person avoid the pain and suffering that I went through than my experience would be worth it.

You will need conviction to follow the same path to a cure. That is why I'm telling my story — to convince you that you need to check yourself out with a specific type of qualified doctor who has a high probability of solving your problem.

If you are reading this book you probably have been examined by professionals. I'll be that you've been X-Rayed, CAT-Scanned, MRI'd and now you are medicated trying to control the pain.

In a sense this is good. Professionals have been running their "playbook" on your condition. They've eliminated the obvious while narrowing the possibilities. Now you still need to find the problem because they have not been able to.

You will not find a magic elixir in here. Instead I will share my experience in overcoming this painful condition. What you will find here is the ability to pre-qualify yourself for a treatment plan that could lead to your recovery. Inside the plan is detailed including the reasoning behind each step. Finally you will also find a valuable referral that will start you on your way.

Your "engine" hasn't been running just right. Up to now you've been going to doctors who are the equivalent of the brake shop, muffler shop, and tire shop. The most important thing that you need to do now is to get in front of the right specialist in order to solve your problem. Come on in and let me show you where the guy with the screwdriver is working.

INTRODUCTION

There are many books on the market to help you "manage your pain," "cope with your pain" and "live with fibromyalgia." This is not one of those books, and if that is what you are looking for I suggest trying the local bookstore or the Internet instead. When I had fibromyalgia I wasn't interested in coping with anything. The only thing I wanted to do was to get *rid* of it!

Yes, fibromyalgia is painful and debilitating. But I don't believe that you should live with it. Why should you? This book is my story about how I was diagnosed with fibromyalgia, and then dared to ask the most important question about it — "Why?" — and then persevered to find a cure.

Now there is something you don't read about very often. A cure for fibromyalgia! The condition is so painful that we tend to concentrate on pain management rather than on finding the cause and fixing it. It is human nature to do so. It is difficult for the fibromyalgia patient to do any more than that because of the immense amount of pain he or she endures.

I want to help you, and I think that just maybe I can. I feel that I have something to offer both fibromyalgia patients and medical professionals. Through a freak accident I experienced the whole spectrum of injury, misdiagnosis, and misguided treatment related to fibromyalgia, followed by — finally — a remarkable recovery, and all within a relatively short period of time. Considering that fibromyalgia and its close cousins, chronic fatigue syndrome and chronic depression, supposedly have no real explanation and no real cure — at least, according to mainstream medicine — I think that my experience can help to shed much-needed light on the problem.

I am not a doctor. I am a layman sharing my experience in terms the average person can understand and relate to. I was diagnosed with fibromyalgia and I overcame it. At one point I was so debilitated that it took two hands and all my strength to painfully lift a dinner plate. Now I lift plates eight at a time with one hand. I no longer take medications to control pain. I don't *need* it.

I think this experience puts me in a rare club. But I present this information on an informational basis only. Please consult a licensed medical practitioner before engaging in treatment for any medical condition. Under the laws of the United States, only a licensed medical practitioner can recommend treatment. I also want to stress that I am not affiliated with nor compensated in any way by any of the organizations mentioned in this book. Rather, I am sharing this information with you solely because I feel that if my story helps just one more person to recover, then it gives purpose to the suffering I personally endured.

Although I have used some medical terminology in this book, I have tried not to get too technical. Most people don't want to learn all of the details about their illness; they just want to get better. So I have provided enough information to help you through the process without boring you with the details. There are plenty of other books filled with the minutiae if you are inclined to read about it. Unfortunately, most books deal with how to cope with fibromyalgia but offer no clues on how to get rid of it. So the focus here will be on the steps you can take to rid yourself of your condition.

Fibromyalgia is a condition much in need of "connecting the dots." I am a special case — I know what caused my fibromyalgia condition, and I know what fixed it. I have provided details about the trail of symptoms that I personally exhibited. These symptoms are not a complete list of possible fibromyalgia symptoms, but are broad enough for you to relate to if you have this condition. I also list the drugs I was given in an attempt to treat the condition. You should be aware that drugs are used to try to treat symptoms of the condition, but have no curative powers. I also took notes during my struggle. At the time I kept those notes to help me reason out what was happening to me, and now they are useful for telling this story.

Plain and simple, fibromyalgia is a condition of the nervous system. Is it any wonder that in the modern world the human nervous system is increasingly "choosing" to refuse to function? Just think of the stress driving alone puts on your body. The human body was not designed to be whipped down the road at 70 miles per hour while being bombarded by the scenery rushing by, nor by the forces at work when the brake is applied. Traffic at rush hour? No stress there! Car accidents, roller coasters, the stress of playing sports, the bombardment of stimuli from television all play an active part in wearing down the natural abilities of the human nervous system to function. And of course, there's the stress experienced from sitting in meetings at work, applying for a job, meeting deadlines, and dealing with all the other daily tribulations of living in today's world.

The more you think about it, it's a wonder that the human nervous system functions at all in this hectic environment. Since your nervous system controls every action in your body, from heart rate to blood pressure to breathing, when your nervous system decides to call in sick it is the sort of thing that can ruin not only your day, but your whole life. When the nervous system checks out, you can count on panic attacks, depression, short temper, mood swings, intolerance to exercise, shooting pain, numbness, tingly sensations, erratic heartbeat, and incontinence. You'll feel cold, then hot. You may also experience a host of other strangely conflicting symptoms that will drive both you and your physician crazy.

Modern medicine is not sure what fibromyalgia is or what causes it. However, it is caused by something; it didn't "just happen." Having experienced this debilitating condition myself, I think that I can shed some light on the subject. I think that fibromyalgia is a condition that is the equivalent of short circuiting your nervous system.

Here's why. Think of your central nervous system as a four-lane freeway. The traffic flowing on the road represents the nerve impulses telling different parts of your body what to feel and how to act. The exit ramps represent nerve attachments to the various body parts, such as your hands, feet, and eyes. Everything flows well on the highway until a worker sets up construction barrels, reduces the traffic to one lane, and blocks exits. This is the condition of your nervous system when you are diagnosed with fibromyalgia.

Enter the physician who has been trained to identify and treat symptoms. Since so many of the "exits" are blocked, the multitude of symptoms confuse him (or her — no sexism intended). He attempts to treat each individual by isolating the symptoms in the manner he was trained to do. He carefully will try this or try that until he finds something that works. Unfortunately, it soon becomes painfully obvious that no single treatment can overcome the multitude of problems.

So finally, after trying to treat your symptoms with painkillers, muscle relaxers, anti-depressants, and myriad other drugs, the confused and exhausted physician gives up and leaves you in a drugged stupor with the bad news: You have fibromyalgia. The drug companies now have medications designed precisely for this condition, so you are given those drugs and then you're told to go home and have a nice life.

This is exactly what happened to me. That was the diagnosis I received after consulting 14 medical professionals. But before I go any further, I want to make an important point. This is my fibromyalgia story. I will be telling you how my nervous system was damaged and the path I took to fix it. Your story may be, and could be, different. What I want to provide you with is enlightenment so you are open to possible causes of your condition, then suggest where you might go, first to diagnose and then to overcome your own physical problem. This process will still involve using professional health care services, although they may not be the ones you are accustomed to using.

If you are not open to new suggestions, just keep doing what you have been. After all, that has been working so well for you! But if you want to overcome your situation, take a fresh look at your problem, and attack it from a different direction, then you have come to the right place.

Please take note. The assumption here is that the reader is suffering from "chronic pain from an unknown origin." Many of the symptoms of fibromyalgia mimic that of other conditions. If you have not previously consulted a licensed physician you should do so immediately. This information is intended for those who have already consulted traditional medical resources and have been unable to obtain a resolution of their problem.

As I mentioned before, I am not a doctor, although after what I have been through I feel like one. I cannot treat you or prescribe anything for you like a doctor can. But I can get you to look at your problem from a different angle and perhaps help you out in that manner. I think that I can point you in the right direction. If you need those medications to help you function, go ahead and take them. But in the meantime, let's take a journey now that just may shed some new light on your old problem.

CHAPTER 1. Get a Bucket of Chicken, Have a Barrel of Fun

What a beautiful autumn day it was that fine October. The sun was shining, the leaves were turning glorious colors, and there was the fresh scent of a crisp fall day. When a coworker asked me to go to lunch, I had no idea that my life was about to change drastically. Let me be clear: I do not blame the Colonel for what happened to me that fateful day. It wasn't his fault that when I visited one of his restaurants that the chickens weren't the only ones that got "winged." In retrospect I think it is safe to say that the experience was far from "a barrel of fun."

To be fair to the Colonel, my back had been hurting me on and off for years. Typically I would go to the doctor and he would prescribe muscle relaxers and painkillers and the ache in my back would go away for a few months. More recently, I had been taking over-the-counter painkillers on a daily basis, and never thought much about it. This enabled me to go to work because it dulled the ache. I was uncomfortable on long car rides, but I dismissed this as just getting older. After all, it had been eight years since my 40th birthday, and some wear and tear was normal. Or at least that was what I thought.

Then I started getting shooting pains in my arms and legs. That kind of pain can be a warning signal, so I was referred to a cardiologist. But after all the tests he could find nothing wrong. Those pains would occur at strange times and for no apparent reason. It didn't happen often enough to stop me from functioning, but rather just often enough to make me wonder what was wrong. No explanation was ever offered by the medical practitioners.

But back to that beautiful fall day. My colleague and I arrived at the local KFC restaurant. I was in the front passenger seat of my coworker's VW Beetle, and I struggled a bit to get out of the car. Unfortunately, with the odd twist I had to make to get out of the car, I didn't notice that we had parked next to a manhole cover, which was an inch or so lower than the pavement. I stepped right onto the cover. That odd drop combined with the twisting motion I made getting out of the car caused something to "pop" in my upper back.

I straightened out, felt slightly flushed, and thought little of it. That is, until we reached the door of the restaurant and I realized that my heart was racing. By the time I sat down at the table I was struggling to walk. I slumped into a chair with both hands tingling. I cut the lunch short and made a hasty retreat back to the office. I told my employees that I was leaving early, and with my heart still pounding, I left the building.

My instinct was that something was "out of place" and that I should see my chiropractor. I did have a chiropractor at the time, a fine doctor I had been seeing for a couple of years. He had been doing the traditional work on my back—the "slamming" adjustments, and the turning and twisting of the body and neck. None of it had been particularly effective, but I was confident that if I were to stay with it long enough then things would get better and my previous mysterious symptoms would disappear.

By the time I reached the chiropractor's office, I was in severe pain. There was numbness and tingling in both arms and my heart was pounding in my ears. I struggled to get into the examining room, and after a consultation, the doctor concluded that because of the pain I was experiencing, I must have broken something. He decided not to touch me, but rather sent me directly to a clinic for X-rays.

When I arrived at the clinic, I was so debilitated that I needed assistance to get up on the table so the pictures could be taken. It was then that the thought occurred to me that whatever was wrong, this was not going to be a simple fix. I moaned in pain as the technician turned me this way and that way, and I was more than relieved when the process ended.

By the next morning the pain had intensified so much that I could barely get out of bed. I struggled to dress, and was glad when the phone rang and my chiropractor was on the other end.

"Great news!" he said enthusiastically. "The X-rays are fine — there's nothing broken or out of place!"

He suggested I take it easy for a few days and see how things "settled down." I would have liked to do just that, but I was still concerned so I summoned my remaining energy and drove over to my long-time family doctor for a consultation. After I explained the pain I was in, my family doctor intently listened to my heart. He clocked it at 140 beats per minute. My resting heart rate would normally be about 65 beats per minute. Typically 140 beats would be about right if I was running on a treadmill. Then he examined my back and calmly stated, "Well, here is your problem: the C-6 vertebra is sticking out!"

The C-6 vertebra is a spinal disc just below the neck in the upper back. He chuckled and instructed me to lie down on the table. Relieved he had found the problem, I gladly did as told and then he "adjusted" the vertebra. He carefully pushed it back into place, and immediately I could feel my heart rate slowing down.

He then performed a chiropractic neck adjustment in which he rotated my head to the left until it cracked and to the right the same way. I stood up and everything felt great. A little dazed by the experience, I was just glad it was something simple. I was instructed to go home and rest.

The next day when I woke up it was a whole new world for me. I was in excruciating pain and was almost unable to move. What lay ahead of me wasn't simple at all.

CHAPTER 2. Could Things Get Any Worse?

I awoke that morning to severe pain in my head, neck, and shoulders. Every movement resulted in pains shooting down my limbs. There was barely enough energy in my body for me to find the motivation for another trip to the physician but I still managed to drag myself back to the doctor's office again.

Unbelievably, he recommended rest. Period. He assured me I would feel better if I just took a few days to relax. He gave me the standard array of muscle relaxers and painkillers to help me feel better. We started to talk about what now seemed to me to be a chronic back condition. I asked the question, "We seem to be going in circles with this. What can I do to get past this? What do other people do?" He assured me that many people have back issues, and that the best thing to do was to get physical therapy (PT). He took out his prescription pad and wrote the name of a local physical therapist, along with "assess and treat" as the prescribed fix for my condition.

As poorly as I felt, I couldn't wait to get some PT and finally put this problem behind me. Even though I wasn't exactly sure what PT was, I still had confidence in standard medical procedures. So when I entered the clinic, I was more than happy to do exactly what the therapist asked me to do.

Now again, I'm no specialist in PT, either, but based on what was done to me, it seems that PT is an attempt to work the body through pain using various techniques to loosen up the muscles. Physical therapists seem to subscribe to the "no pain, no gain" philosophy. They prescribed a routine of pulling on some bungee ropes and lifting some small weights. Then the therapist applied heat while pulling and turning various parts of my neck and body. Combining the heat with the medication I was taking felt very good, and when I went home I was encouraged by the experience.

But when I woke up the next day, I was in even more pain, so much pain that I was unable to move an inch without excruciating pain radiating throughout my body. I struggled to get out of bed, and fortunately, it seemed that as I moved things "loosened up." Tears fell from my eyes as I put my clothes on—dressing was now a painful experience, too.

I returned for a second day of physical therapy. The therapist repeated the same process as before. That night, I was in too much pain to walk to the bedroom so I slept on the floor in the family room. When I woke up, I would say the pain level was so high that I would classify my condition as totally debilitated and incapacitated. It was a major effort to walk to the bathroom, and when I arrived I was exhausted.

I decided to return to the physical therapist and tell him what was happening. He assured me that I should continue "treatment," and that things would improve. But I said I couldn't because I had pain shooting throughout my body. He argued that wasn't unusual and that with work the pain would go away. I had to sit while discussing the situation because I was shaking and didn't have the energy left to stand. He told me to go over to the bungee ropes and start pulling. I pulled just once and pain shot up my arm and into my head. Nauseous, I dropped the ropes, and as I slowly and painfully made my way to the door he pleaded with me to come back and continue. I told him I was going to go in a different direction.

CHAPTER 3. Where Does It Hurt?

At this point, when I returned to my family doctor, I knew I had a serious problem. My condition was keeping me from work—in fact, a return to work seemed very far away. I explained to him that with the level of pain I was experiencing something had to be broken. Maybe I didn't look like I was in pain, because he seemed rather skeptical. Even though he was somewhat reluctant, I talked him into doing some testing. He told me that he thought this was a muscular issue and that nothing would show up in the tests. He set up an appointment for an MRI and a bone scan. The soonest I could get the appointment was two painful days later.

By the morning of the appointment I was no longer able to drive on my own. My wife had to help me out to the car. By this time I had tremendous pain in my neck and any movement whatsoever would increase the discomfort. While in the car, I could feel every bump in the road, and I sat in silence cringing with every thump of the tires on the road. When we finally arrived at the clinic, my wife dropped me off at the door and then parked the car. I barely had enough energy to walk into the lobby.

The bone scan was simple enough. I was eager to have it done, sure that some major component of my neck or spine had to be broken. I knew that the technician could not tell me if there was a problem, but I had enough previous encounters with technicians to know that even the technician can see major issues. She gave me the usual disclaimers and then showed me my scan on the computer monitor. "This looks great!" she exclaimed. "See how straight everything is!"

When I went back out to the front desk I asked when the MRI was scheduled. The receptionist checked her book and said the earliest available appointment would be in two weeks. Up until this point I had been relatively calm. I am a patient person. But the pain was so intense that I couldn't take it anymore. I started gesturing wildly and screaming at her that I was in unbelievable pain and that I needed an MRI *stat!* Flustered by my outburst, she checked her schedule again and told me if I cared to wait until the end of the day they would fit me in last.

I agreed and sat in the lobby for five painful hours holding my neck with one arm, because the pressure seemed to help the pain. At one point, no doubt feeling sympathetic, the receptionist came out and asked me if my doctor had been giving me anything for the pain. I explained that the pain I felt was coming right through with the painkillers. She cringed and returned to the reception desk.

The MRI technician gave no clue as to the results of the test. But I felt better knowing that I had undergone two tests that should reveal the extent of the internal damage. I was prepared mentally for some surgery to fix what I thought must be a broken neck.

Two days later I summoned all of my remaining strength to return to my family doctor, where I sat in the examination room holding up my head with my arm because I could barely lift it otherwise. My physician had taken good care of me for more than 25 years. We had been through adult-onset chicken pox, pneumonia, several bouts of sinus infections, and numerous other afflictions over the years. I can't say enough about the quality of my family doctor. He was always there for me, and would take the time to talk with me about whatever my ailment might be.

But I was about to see a side of medicine that I had never witnessed before. My doctor came into the examination room, and after dispensing with the usual pleasantries, we started discussing my situation. He gave a strange look at me, sitting there holding my head up with one hand, but it didn't seem to concern him at the moment. He looked through the test results. "No anomaly" was checked off on every box on the form. "Good news," he said. "Nothing is broken or out of place."

He looked at me studying my head and neck. He seemed somewhat amused that I was holding my head up with my arm. He didn't appear to grasp the difficulty I was having just sitting in front of him. After a few reflective moments, he tried to diagnose the root of my problem when he asked the question I will never forget: "Where does it hurt?"

On the surface, this would not seem to be such a difficult question. For instance, if you fall and injure your hand, then you explain that the hand hurts. This directs the physician to your hand, as opposed to, say, your arm. It is a simple diagnostic question that we have all been asked at one time or another. How tough can it be? But I stared back at him in silence. As odd as it might seem, I was unable to answer the question.

He looked at me inquisitively. Maybe thinking I hadn't heard him the first time, he asked again, "Where is the pain the greatest? Where does it hurt the most?"

I was deep in thought at that moment, and finally broke the silence. "I don't know, I can't answer that question."

He raised an eyebrow and looked at me with a puzzled expression. I couldn't put into words the pain that I was feeling. It radiated throughout my entire body. It also didn't originate from anywhere in particular, but rather seemed to come from everywhere.

I knew I had to offer something. How could he fix this if I can't even tell him where it hurts? I was a college graduate without a vocabulary equipped to address the situation. The pain was intense, indescribable. "I'll tell you what," I offered. "I'll tell you where it doesn't hurt."

That seemed reasonable to him, and he nodded his head in approval. So I paused for a moment to consider where it didn't hurt. He looked stunned when I gave my answer: "My eyebrows— they don't hurt."

I had nothing else to offer. I think he thought I was joking. I wasn't. I also think he thought I was crazy.

After a few moments of consideration he shrugged his shoulders. He explained that he had never seen a case like mine before, and didn't know what to do with me. He suggested that I go home and rest. I said that was unacceptable; that I needed to know what was wrong. He told me he didn't know.

When I pressed him to give me a diagnosis after all of the testing he had done, he finally said, "You have fibromyalgia. Pain throughout the body for no known reason." He wrote, "Fibromyalgia, treat with rest," on a prescription pad.

"How long would you like to be out of work?" he asked next. I told him I didn't need that because I thought my employer would be understanding, so I left with only the note.

I didn't know it then, but that was just the start of my journey.

CHAPTER 4. Always Get a Second Opinion

It helped to have a label for my condition. At least I could spend time researching fibromyalgia. But most of what I found was bleak. Essentially fibromyalgia is a default diagnosis—meaning that you have unexplained pain. According to WebMD there are more than 5 million people with fibromyalgia, most of them women, in the United States. Most people never recover. Essentially, patients are told to go home and learn how to cope and live with the pain.

Six weeks passed, and it was apparent rest wasn't going to help anything. My family doctor had exhausted all known options concerning what was causing my problem. I continued to deteriorate on a daily basis. At that point, I walked slowly and was stooped over like a 100-year-old man. In fact, I've seen 100-year-old men move quicker and with more energy than I had. My hands shook, and my body hurt from head to toe. I asked my doctor where I could get a neck brace to help hold my head up. My doctor wrote out a prescription for me. I never did get it filled, though. I didn't have the energy to go to the medical store to buy it.

My doctor admitted that he must be missing something, and suggested I get a second opinion. I told him that I didn't really have anyplace else to go, so he took out his prescription pad and wrote down a name and a number. I couldn't believe my longtime, trusted doctor had come to this—he had essentially thrown his hands up and given up!

I had always heard that whenever you had a serious medical problem it was a good idea to get a second opinion. It makes good sense. Again I summoned up all my energy for a trip to a clinic to see another M.D. named Dr. Hubris (not his real name). Again I was unable to drive myself, so my wife drove me to the appointment. She parked right outside the door and I struggled to walk just a few feet into the office and sit down.

I was handed a clipboard and a multi-page information sheet. I took the pen in my hand and tried to write my name. I couldn't do it because my hand was shaking so violently. I had to hand the clipboard to my wife and have her complete the forms for me.

While you don't know Dr. Hubris, if you have seen the program "House" on TV, then you know exactly what he is like. I waited for an hour for an audience with him, and he strutted into the examination room exuding arrogance and self-importance. Normally a person with this sort of personality makes an entrance on top of an elephant, but I supposed the ceiling was too low in the clinic to fit one in. Apparently they teach Egotism 101 in med school, and Dr. Hubris had aced it. To call him pompous would be kind. I guess I was supposed to be honored to be in his presence. I wasn't.

He did seem knowledgeable, though, and after performing a thorough examination that included taking blood and urine samples, and doing a thorough examination of my neck and spine, he decided that what I needed was steroids, painkillers, muscle relaxers, and more PT. In my worn-down mental state it seemed reasonable at the time, although today I don't know why. I allowed him to inject me with the steroids. He called ahead to another physical therapist and I went straight from the clinic to PT.

The PT office was located in the basement of a medical building. At this point, I was unable to walk down a flight of stairs so I was relieved that they had an elevator. This therapist seemed incredibly intelligent and seemed to grasp my situation. I was excited that I had finally found the "A" team of professionals I needed to help fix my broken body. The therapist gently interviewed me and then decided upon a treatment regimen.

Essentially, a physical therapist works the muscular system. The theory is that by strengthening muscles, the bones will come back into alignment and one's health will improve. People with tired and worn-out muscles go to PT to be rejuvenated by a series of heat treatments, stretching, and weight exercises. The course of treatment this therapist described was different from that of the first PT and seemed to fit my case.

One morning, after several PT visits, I noticed in the mirror that my shoulders were not "squared up." Instead, one shoulder was lower than the other. At the time, I laughed to myself, thinking, "Well, there is the problem right there!" I mentioned it to the therapist and he looked at me and remarked, "Don't worry about that, it happens all the time." Because of his reassurances, I thought little of it after that.

My condition seemed to improve slowly. At least until the drugs ran out. Then within a three-day period I went from functioning at a minimal level to a new low. On December 23, 2006, three months after the onset of symptoms, I was sitting on a machine slowly working my arms when pains started shooting down all my limbs and the room started to spin. My ears started popping and I saw flashes of light. I could feel a panic attack beginning to start up — yet another thing that had started happening to me at random since the onset of my injury. I stopped exercising, summoned my remaining strength, and simply walked out. Maybe staggered out would be a more accurate description. The receptionist yelled at me to come back, but I ignored her and continued outside into a freezing rain.

My symptoms now included intolerance to the cold. I was bundled up in a jacket with gloves and a hat yet was shivering in the outside temperature. I had a follow-up appointment with Dr. Hubris scheduled right after the PT, so I drove the few blocks to his clinic, then sat in the car for an hour as the rain drummed on the roof, waiting for the clinic to open.

By the time the door opened at 11 a.m., I was shaking uncontrollably and blinking back tears brought on by the pain. True to his usual schedule, I had to sit in the lobby for another hour before Dr. Hubris graced me with his presence, fully an hour late for my appointment.

In the examination room, Dr. Hubris took one look at me and then left the room. He returned carrying a box of tissues. He handed it to me and said, "Here, you are going to need this."

I was puzzled by the statement, but took the box from him. Standing in front of me, he explained that many people get depressed at Christmas time. He asked how my job was going, and I told him not really all that well because I was unable to work. After all, I was in so much pain I could barely concentrate on anything, so work was impossible.

He then told me that he thought I was faking my condition and trying to get on disability, and that he would not authorize it. Instead, he took out his prescription pad, and wrote down the name and number of a psychiatrist, saying I should seek out psychological help because there was nothing else he could do for me.

Apparently satisfied by the great job he had done with his expert diagnosis he turned his back on me and triumphantly strutted out of the room in a grand flurry of ego. All he needed was a trumpet fanfare and a feathered cap. Yes, the circus had left town!

I sat for a few minutes in the exam room, stunned by what had occurred. The receptionist broke the silence by entering and telling me that they needed the room, and asked if I would be so kind as to leave. Far be it for me to get in the way of misdiagnosing more patients, so completely demoralized, I gingerly stood up and slowly returned to my car.

The moral of the Dr. Hubris story is: Always get a second opinion on your medical condition, but don't be surprised at what you find. (I will say, though, that I sincerely hope your second opinion goes better than mine did.) The good news is it was Dr. Hubris's incredibly pathetic diagnosis and pompous, cavalier attitude towards my severe pain that served as my motivation to write this book and possibly help others avoid the problems I encountered during my quest to recover.

Don't be surprised if your condition is greeted with the same enthusiasm that I encountered with Dr. Hubris. Given my own experience, I am pretty sure that there are many other people out there who are doomed by the same mainstream medical "treatment" I encountered.

If anything else good came out of my experience with Dr. Hubris, it was this: At long last, the wind was about to change direction just for me.

CHAPTER 5. Christmas Epiphany

It was Christmas Day 2006. The night before, I had visited the in-laws for Christmas Eve dinner. While sitting at the table, I used my right hand to hold myself upright by grasping the edge of the table. As the merriment around me continued I was lost in a world of pain wondering how I was ever going to overcome my situation. Nobody seemed to notice the condition I was in, I'm sure I just sat staring off into space.

The following morning at home on Christmas Day, while entertaining my side of the family, I was again holding onto the table in same manner while everyone around me was talking and generally making merry. My hands shook as I ate and at least once I dropped my fork because my hand was unable to grasp and hold it.

It was that moment that something basic but intuitive occurred to me. I could picture in my mind all of the doctors and therapists who had been treating me. They were all home with their families enjoying Christmas dinner. None of them were thinking about me. But here I was, with my life on hold, writhing in pain at the most joyous time of the year.

It was clear that the traditional medical profession had failed me. Various experienced and learned medical professionals had examined, tested, and imaged me to the best of their ability. Since their methodology did not provide any positive results, they concluded that no problem existed and that the patient must be okay. In an odd backwards sense, this was a logical conclusion. The problem was, of course, that I wasn't okay. I was in severe, debilitating pain that was getting progressively worse.

As Albert Einstein said, "Insanity is doing the same thing over and over again and expecting to get different results." That described the insanity I was experiencing perfectly, and I realized that going to see another traditional doctor was not a reasonable option. I decided that if I was ever going to get better, I was going to have to abandon traditional medical channels and go in a different direction. Somehow, I was going to have to find a way to think differently and find a solution on my own to my problem. I also realized that the solution was not going to be found at the pharmacy or in a traditional medical clinic.

I wasn't in a condition to do much of anything, so I spent my time pondering what I should do next. Among other things, I began looking on the Internet, searching online and looking at diagrams of the body, trying to determine what could be causing the symptoms I was experiencing. I even kept the prescription for the psychiatrist in front of my monitor and used it as motivation to help me overcome my problems myself. I knew I was not insane, but the doctors were making me feel like I was. My pain was real, but they didn't believe that it was real. So how could they find out what was wrong if they weren't even making an attempt to look?

I decided that I wasn't going to wait around any longer for the medical community to figure me out. It became my personal mission to be my own health advocate and solve the mystery on my own. Not to mention, I figured there would be a lot of personal satisfaction in proving that Dr. Hubris was an idiot. That thought alone kept me going through the pain.

CHAPTER 6. Divine Intervention

Having decided to take my fate into my own hands, the obvious question was what to do next. Searching the Internet had yielded no answers. Frankly, I had no idea what to do now. So I decided to rest and further ponder my fate. At that point I was no longer going to work, and I would spend the day seated in a recliner in pain. I could do little more than use the remote control to change the channels on the television, and even then I would usually fall asleep within minutes of turning the TV on. Using the bathroom was a chore. It would take all of my strength and energy to rise out of the chair and shuffle across the house. When I would return to my chair, I would be exhausted from the effort and would fall asleep immediately.

I tried reading to pass the time. Since I could not hold my head up or even hold a book in my hands, I would lie in bed on my stomach and hold the book over the edge as I scanned a page. I usually fell asleep immediately after reading a few paragraphs. I had heard about chronic fatigue syndrome, depression, and fibromyalgia, and it was occurring to me that I might be suffering from all of these.

Even my brain seemed to be moving in slow motion. When watching TV I could barely keep up with the action on the set. Any kind of loud noise would set my hearting pounding for hours and trigger a smashing headache. I was having difficulty talking because I could not think of words fast enough to complete a sentence. I would pause in the middle of a sentence and lose my train of thought, forgetting what I was discussing. It hurt to take a deep breath. Bright light caused headaches. I spent hours with the blinds closed just sitting in the dark and trying not to move.

They say when you are near death that your life flashes before you. In an eerie twist, when I would sit quietly my life would start to scroll by slowly. I could see myself in grade school talking to someone as though it was happening at that moment. I could look around the classroom as though I was still sitting in it. I could reflect on moments in my life that occurred years earlier as they slowly made their way across the screen in my mind, with all of the details were vividly intact. The slow-motion parade continued for weeks every time I closed my eyes.

The thought occurred to me that if this was how I was going to live I didn't want to go on. I tried to free my soul to let go and leave it all behind. I was clinging so feebly to life that it seemed as though that thought alone would set me free. But as soon as the thought occurred to me, a mysterious voice spoke loudly and clearly in my head, causing both of my ears to hurt from the vibration. It said, "It is not your time yet."

I was somewhat taken by surprise at this pronouncement, and to this day, I dare not speculate on where the voice came from. But this encouragement helped me to look past the depression and look ahead to a better future.

Even so, one thing was for sure: I continued to be confused about what to do next. I was still contemplating my next move when "funny things" began happening to my vision. I would see bright flashes and little helicopter-like things spinning, accompanied by massive headaches. My eyes were sensitive to light, and when the lights in a room would go out it would take several minutes for my eyes to adjust to the dark. My vision was "foggy," like I was like looking through a heavy white fog even though my surroundings were clear. This effect would come and go on a random basis. It was a scary situation, and I thought I was going blind on top of all of the other things that were happening to me.

I decided to visit my eye doctor to get the grim news. Who would think, very oddly, in this bizarre journey that another turning point in my condition would occur when I visited the eye doctor?

Dr. Becker earned her degree in England. As part of her training she was required to work in a psychiatric ward. As she checked my vision, I relayed my story to her. She told me one of the things that she had learned in the psychiatric ward was that women often suffered depression, but not so much because they had serious physical problems. Rather, the reason generally was that they were often unable to convince a doctor that they had a problem. Their symptoms were dismissed as "imagination," and the sense of hopelessness that set in would lead to depression and often to suicide.

You may find it interesting to know that more than 90% of fibromyalgia cases occur in women. Doctors often mistakenly dismiss their symptoms as "emotional female issues" and then women sufferers have their situation compounded by the same dynamics Dr. Becker described. There is a certain amount of disbelief that the condition is "real" and this also hinders treatment.

I think the high percentage of female sufferers is easy to explain. As you will see, my hypothesis is that fibromyalgia is the result of a physically damaged central nervous system. I will elaborate more on this later. It follows that women would have more trouble with the nervous system than men. The muscular/skeletal construction of the (typical) female body is simply more prone to injury than the (typically) more muscular male structure. The finer bone density and muscle mass of a female make her more prone to injury.

This is not a sexist remark, but rather a simple observation about the height and weight of the average female versus the average male. Since it takes more of a "jolt" to damage the male structure, it follows that fewer men would be injured due to an accident or wear and tear in the spinal region.

But back to Dr. Becker. She carefully examined my eyes, and thoughtfully tried not to have me turn my head too much in the process. She could tell I was in pain and made every effort not to aggravate the injury — in short, she was far more sympathetic to my plight than any of the other medical professionals I had consulted. Dr. Becker explained to me that I was experiencing migraine headaches — which, by the way, are another symptom of a central nervous system problem.

She surmised that much of what was ailing me was "anomalies of the central nervous system" and that my condition should improve with time. She also told me that the trick was to get in front of the right professional, and that when I did things would work out. She encouraged me not to get discouraged and to keep looking until I found the right professional to help me recover.

To this day I credit Dr. Becker's diagnosis as a major turning point in my recovery. Her words rang true for me, and made me realize that the feelings of depression I had been experiencing were not a result of my condition, but rather the hopelessness that had set in as a result of not finding the right professionals to help me. I also realized that although I definitely was depressed, the drugs I was taking did not cause that depression, nor did my depression cause fibromyalgia as some professionals had insinuated.

So removing my depression was not going to cure me. No, I was depressed because I had fibromyalgia, and my life was on hold because I was held hostage by my painful condition. This is counter to prevailing thinking on fibromyalgia – the mainstream thought is that somehow depression causes the problem.

These thoughts helped me through this difficult time. It was this "second wind" that enabled me to continue my search on my own for a cure for my condition, and eventually resulted in finding the health care team that helped me recover at last.

But I'm getting ahead of myself. I spent the next few months resting with little improvement. By this time, my employer was getting impatient and no longer called to see how I was doing. By April 2007, I was hanging on by a thread. I had lost 50 pounds, mostly because I didn't have the energy to get off the chair and walk to the kitchen, a distance of less than 10 feet. Worse yet, I was still unsure about my next move.

Now here is perhaps the strangest and fortuitous part of my story. Inexplicably one April morning in 2007 I rose from that easy chair and went over to the kitchen table. I decided I wanted to read the newspaper. I had not been able to read for some time, and honestly had not looked at the newspaper since the previous October. I ignored the front page and Section B, and opened to the sports section instead. I read a couple of paragraphs on the front page of the sports section, and turned the page twice more looking for something more interesting.

That was when I saw the advertisement, which shone like a beacon. It read, "Doctor has success with fibromyalgia patients." The doctor referred to was a chiropractor who used a "gentle method" to treat patients. I really don't know what appealed to me about the advertisement. Normally I dismiss this sort of thing as just a marketing technique designed to get you to spend money. But this advertisement intrigued me, and since it offered an initial consultation for a mere $25, I figured I had nothing to lose so I might as well try it.

There are two points worth mentioning here. The first is that this was the only newspaper I had looked at in more than six months. I read just two paragraphs in two different articles in the paper that that fateful day, as well as the advertisement itself. Having read only those things, I was exhausted and unable to read further. The second point is that the advertisement for Dr. Rich was the only printed advertisement he had placed in the entire year, and it appeared in the newspaper only on that day! Surely providence was at work here.

I made an appointment for May 1, 2007. That morning I felt so bad I was torn between keeping the appointment or heading to a medical supply store to buy a wheelchair so I could get around a bit more. I did not have enough energy to drive very far, so I opted to make the painful journey to see Dr. Rich because his office was closer to my home than the medical supply store.

I parked as close to the door of the medical building as possible and shuffled painfully to the elevator. The slow rise of the elevator to the second floor aggravated the pain in my neck and shoulder and I winced in pain when it stopped at the second floor. In Dr. Rich's office, I slumped into a chair. I scribbled my way through the forms I was given and tiredly waited for help.

The examination was thorough but not really that long. I told Dr. Rich that I felt like I was 100 years old and if the wind blew too hard I would simply crumple to the ground in a heap. Dr. Rich took measurements of my spine and noted that my shoulders were not straight, as I personally had observed months earlier. My left shoulder was three inches higher than my right. The most painful part of the examination was the X-rays. I was in so much pain that I had to be helped up onto the table. Dr. Rich took only a few shots, and I noticed that they were not taken at the same angles as any of the previous X-rays had been taken.

Eventually, he put the developed photos up on an X-ray illuminator and invited me to come over and look. He announced with a somewhat grim look that he had both good news and bad news. I asked for the bad news first, so he pointed to the pictures and explained that we were looking down and sideways at the atlas, which is the topmost vertebra in the spine. In medical parlance, it's the C-1 vertebra, and it's the bone on which the base of the brain sits.

Dr. Rich explained that the amount of pain a displaced atlas will cause is related to how many degrees of "tilt" the bone has. As little as a one-degree tilt can cause severe pain. He showed how mine was crooked by six degrees. Six degrees! It was so plainly evident on the X-ray that this bone was grossly out of place that even I could see it. On another photo we looked down on the discs from the top of the head. Again, even I could see that the discs were not lined up; rather, they were all askew. He grimaced as he pointed to the photos and remarked, "This must really hurt!"

Now, normally I might have responded to that with some sarcastic remark like, "Figure that out all by yourself did you?" But after what I had been through, I was speechless. But more importantly, his remark immediately lifted my spirits, because after all the professionals I had seen and all the imaging that had been done, this was the first time that somebody had pointed to something and said, "See this is your problem right here!"

I don't know why no one else saw what Dr. Rich saw. As I mentioned, his X-rays were taken from different angles than traditional back X-rays, so that may explain it. For whatever reason, everybody else had completely missed the problem and therefore had been unable to diagnose it correctly.

Of course, I asked next what the good news was.

"I can fix this!" he said.

While this was music to my ears, to say I was somewhat skeptical would be an understatement. After all I had been through, I couldn't imagine that somebody could both find the problem and fix it. But he certainly seemed confident, and since I had pretty much exhausted all other options, I was ready to give the treatment a try.

Until this point I had always thought, "A chiropractor is a chiropractor;" that they are all the same. If you take nothing else away from this book, you need to know that there are many different disciplines within the chiropractic profession. I don't pretend to know them all, but I do know that I had stumbled upon something very different that day.

Typically when you think of a chiropractor you think of someone who does a bone-cracking, twisting treatment that sets things straight. Many people are afraid of this kind of treatment. My first chiropractor practiced this method, which is said to be beneficial for the lower back. It should be noted that, according to the Centers for Disease Control and Prevention (CDC, at cdc.gov), 95% of all back problems involve lower back pain.

My pain was the result of a combined upper back and neck injury. This occurs in the other 5% of patients with back problems. Injury in the upper back and neck results in many neurological events throughout the body and can present itself in a variety of ways. Since 95% of back problems are lower back problems, a physician is unlikely to recognize an upper back problem when it's presented to him or her.

Simply put, upper back and neck injury is an "out of the ordinary," low-probability event without specific symptoms. The relative rarity of this type of condition might explain the apparent "disconnect" between treatment of an upper back injury like mine and the approach taken by practitioners of mainstream medicine.

There are certain chiropractors, like Dr. Rich, who *are* trained to recognize this type of out-of-the-ordinary back injury and know how to treat it. They're known as upper cervical chiropractors, meaning that their specialty is working the atlas bone at the top of the spine, as well as the small bones just beneath it all the way down the neck. The "bone cracking" chiropractor does not work this part of the spine; instead, he or she works the lower back and upward toward the mid-back. Conversely, an upper cervical chiropractor works from the top down, the theory being that when things are straight and aligned at the top of the spine the rest of the vertebrae will fall into line. (You can learn more about this specialty and view a video at the website for the National Upper Cervical Chiropractic Association (NUCCA) found at www.nucca.org)

Dr. Rich instructed me to lie on my side on a low table that was more like a padded plank than an exam table. I was terrified, and told him I didn't think I could survive a "bone-cracking experience." He laughed and said that was not how he did things. Once I was in place, he touched the left side of my head just above the ear and then pressed gently. Then he tapped the back of my neck a few times with a small tool that I later learned is called an "activator," which is a small handheld, spring-loaded instrument that looks a little like a plunger. It makes a sound like a stapler when it's applied to the body, and can be used both on bare skin and through clothing (and even shoes).

I have to admit that my first thought after undergoing this simple adjustment was that this was some sort of quackery. Dr. Rich seemingly hadn't done anything except lean on the side of my head and tap lightly on my neck, a process that took no more than a couple of minutes. I couldn't imagine what he could possibly have accomplished.

As I sat up, I thought that I would be leaving and never coming back to see this "quack." But I was soon amazed to discover that my head felt better! I can't describe the sensation; it was as though Dr. Rich had reached inside of me and touched some broken part for the first time — and made it feel better. It was quickly apparent that this was not chicanery, but rather it was very good science at work.

That was the start of my recovery. For those expecting a miracle cure I don't want to oversell my experience. This was the first treatment in a course of treatment hat continued for months. *But I felt better immediately*, by, say, 5 or 10%. Over the next few months I continued to return to Dr. Rich, and I continued to improve. It was a slow, gradual process, but there is no question in my mind that the continual straightening of the upper cervical bones caused the improvement that I experienced.

One by one my previous symptoms faded away. For the next 12 months I continued to take over-the-counter Motrin, the only pain reliever that had done any good. After that, I was "drug free." Using an ice pack on the back of the head and neck also provided relief as treatment continued. I kept improving over the next 24 months in stages, which would be followed by periods of no improvement at all.

I learned that nerves take time to heal once they have been traumatized. Even after the pain was reduced, the nerves continued to be irritated. This improved with time, too, and eventually the nerves calmed down. The last step in my recovery was provided by Connie, my massage therapist, who was recommended to me by Doctor Rich.

Connie worked hard to break up the scar tissue that had formed while I was injured and unable to move around. She also helped to reposition nerves that had moved out of place.

On my first trip to the massage therapist I was so traumatized that when Connie touched me it set off a wave of muscle spasms throughout my body. Keep in mind; this was my condition *after* things had been straightened out by the chiropractor. It took several trips to the massage therapist before things finally began to calm down. Again, icing afterwards was a big help staying comfortable after a massage.

So here it is—based on my experience, my theory is that fibromyalgia as well as chronic fatigue syndrome are a result of a physical upper cervical condition. This condition can be relieved with proper adjustment of the spine and rehabilitation of the damaged tissue through massage therapy.

My experience proves that injury or misalignment to the upper spine in the head or neck area can cause a long list of disturbing neurological events, including chronic fatigue and chronic pain. A parade of medical professionals has also proven that this type of injury is difficult to detect unless you know exactly what you are looking for. For some odd reason, injury to this area is often overlooked by mainstream medical practitioners. In my case it took many medical professionals before I found one who could identify the problem.

Misaligned cervical conditions can be caused by many different circumstances. This is generally a slowly deteriorating condition that occurs over time. Activities such as working in front of a computer (my profession!), sedentary desk work, or repetitive bending work (such as performed by a barber, carpet layer, or dentist) can cause deterioration of muscles which leads to misalignment. In addition a jolt to the neck such as from a car accident or amusement park ride can cause things to begin to slowly drift out of place. These small increments of misalignment are barely noticeable but are cumulative in effect.

As a result of my positive experience, I have since referred more than 15 people to Dr. Rich. The results all of these people have experienced have been extraordinary. We joke among ourselves that his technique is similar to Voodoo — it just doesn't seem possible that such low impact treatment could have such a monumental effect. But it does!

CHAPTER 7. The Truth About Fibromyalgia

The prevailing thought on fibromyalgia, perpetuated by evidence-based medicine, is that treating the condition with some magical elixir will cure it. The thought is that some shortage of "something" in the body is causing the problem, and simply restoring whatever it is will result in a cure. However, while you search for the magic elixir you are supposed to manage your pain with more chemicals. You are supposed to live with the problem while this so-called transformation occurs.

In some cases, fibromyalgia may also be called chronic fatigue syndrome or chronic depression, but no matter what it's called, here's what usually happens. You experience pain, you take muscle relaxers and painkillers, and then you have more pain. Next comes more muscle relaxers and stronger painkillers—and even more pain. Then you'll repeat this sequence until debilitating fibromyalgia sets in. Does this sound familiar?

This treatment is the standard accepted regimen to combat fibromyalgia. But please don't blame your physician for this situation. Your physician is only doing what he/she was trained to do as a practitioner of evidence-based medicine, which is to identify symptoms and then treat them. This works fairly well for some conditions, but for fibromyalgia and related conditions it is a recipe for failure, because there is no dosage of drugs that can correct a mechanical misalignment of the bones in your spine.

Motrin, Lyrica, Lodine, Darvocet, Novocain, steroids, Advil, Valium, Rhinocort, and Astelin. I took them all. This is just a partial list of the chemical warfare that was used to combat my condition. Some of this stuff actually made me feel a little bit better for a short time. Of course, treating the symptoms of this dreaded condition with chemicals avoids the most important question, which is: Why are you in pain? What is causing your discomfort? It's important to note here that *none* of these chemicals have any healing properties; they simply bring some comfort by relieving the symptoms you are feeling.

While being treated for fibromyalgia, I was also treated for depression. The theory was that my depression was causing my body to experience extreme fatigue and pain. Yes, I was depressed — who wouldn't be? — but the expectation of clearing up my physical problems by "curing" my depression was simply not logical. As I said before, the depression did not cause my fibromyalgia; the fibromyalgia caused the depression!

Another "symptom" of fibromyalgia is shallow breathing. Doctors look at it as though somehow breathing shallowly can cause this painful condition. Several health care professionals insinuated that getting me to breathe deeply would fix things. What I know is that when I was injured, whenever I took even a medium breath the area behind my rib cage was extremely painful. I learned to control the pain by breathing more shallowly. So in my experience, shallow breathing is an effect of, but not the cause of fibromyalgia. It is this kind of "chicken and the egg" quandary that causes so much misdirection in searching for a cure for fibromyalgia.

Without addressing the underlying reason for your pain, you are simply kicking the can down the road as the condition worsens. By treating the symptoms with drugs you are essentially hoping to feel better on the premise that the condition will clear itself up and go away. Sometimes it will, sometimes it won't.

Generally, however, rest and relaxation *won't* make fibromyalgia go away. It is estimated there are more than 5 million chronic fibromyalgia sufferers in America, and assuming that they're receiving medication and being told to breathe deeply like I was, it's pretty safe to assume that this traditional strategy doesn't work. What we should be asking is if the "magic elixir" strategy works so well, why are there still 5 million sufferers out there?

The most important information you can know about fibromyalgia is that it is a condition, not a virus or a disease. The average person may not initially grasp the importance of this distinction as it relates to fibromyalgia, so it is worth dwelling on. A virus is contagious and is transmitted from person to person, infecting others as it spreads. A disease is a condition that impairs the normal functioning of a part of the body. Both are generally fairly easy to diagnose because they usually have telltale verifiable markers that make them easy to identify. You can be immunized against a virus and given antibiotics or other medication to cure a virus. Modern medicine also has a wide range of effective modalities to treat and cure many common diseases.

But this is not the case with the condition known as fibromyalgia. A condition describes a circumstance or situation of the body. It is not contagious or transferable; rather, it is a state that the body has been put in. This is an important distinction because if a body can be put into a condition due to an accident, overuse injury or any other situation, it follows that it can be taken *out* of that condition, as well. What I'm saying is that in many cases fibromyalgia is a mechanical condition, not a chemical one. Therefore it follows that chemicals will not cure a mechanical condition.

Here's the rub. A condition can be caused by many different circumstances that vary from person to person. This is why there is no single "cure" for fibromyalgia, because any number of things can put your body into this condition. When a physician diagnoses you with fibromyalgia, the physician is only saying, "Here is the situation." The physician will not say how the condition occurred because he or she probably can't say for sure. Since the physician doesn't know what caused the condition it is difficult to say how to resolve it. Despite this, it's interesting to note that seldom will a physician say it is irreversible.

Once the nervous system is stressed in the neck or upper back in any of these ways, it continues to deteriorate. The traumatized nervous system is "overloaded" and has difficulty coping with even mundane events. Simple things such as exposure to light and sound, as well as basic movements add stress and easily overwhelm the damaged system, resulting in strange symptoms.

For instance, at one point I could not handle something as simple as a vehicle tailgating me on the highway. This normally routine annoyance would upset me so much I would get a headache, my heart would race, and I would have to pull off the road and let the vehicle go by or else I would lose my temper. On one occasion, I drove across town, arrived with trembling hands, and then vomited upon exiting the car. These were all symptoms of an underlying nervous system problem, and as my recovery progressed, my reaction to these types of events returned to "normal."

What are some of the known ways to acquire fibromyalgia? According to the CDC, more than likely it is a combination of things that set up the condition. As mentioned previously, my personal experience as well as the experience of others I have encountered indicates that fibromyalgia appears to be a condition of the upper cervical spine that affects the central nervous system.

According to NUCCA, any number of shocks to the spine at various times in your life can predispose the condition to occur, even many years after the event. A blow to the head, neck, or spine; a minor traffic accident; deteriorating muscle tone; repetitive stress, or repetitive motion can all be precursors to the condition. These are exactly the same things that cause atlas misalignment.

Much like the leaning tower of Pisa, the spine slowly, over time, starts to tip, or become misaligned. (This is known as spinal subluxation.) The body tries to adjust but eventually the "lean" becomes severe and painful. Just like the famous tower, the body will need help if it ever is to be straight again.

Here's another way to look at it. Having your spine out of alignment is like having a dislocated shoulder, which must be put back into place in order to heal. Rest, relaxation, and painkillers will not address the underlying problem. The longer you wait to treat a dislocated shoulder, the worse the problem — and the pain — gets. Some people get lucky with a dislocated shoulder and it goes back into place on its own. Most aren't that lucky and need help putting the shoulder back into place.

In the case of a misaligned spine, the trick, of course, is to find the "out of place" joint or joints that are causing the problem so they can be put back into place. For each person, the location in the spine and the symptoms it causes will differ. While the symptoms can be confusing, it is the job of the upper cervical chiropractor to determine which joints are out of place and to gently correct the problem.

There are actually some telltale signs of an upper cervical problem, and you can check yourself right now to see if you have any of them:

First, stand in front of a mirror. Look straight ahead. Is your head straight, or is it tilted to the left or right? People with upper cervical issues often carry their head tilted to one side and have difficulty keeping their head straight.

Next, look at your shoulders. Are they even, or is one shoulder lower than the other?

After that, consider this: Do you get "pinched nerves" in the neck? Numbness or tingling in the fingers or toes? Upper back pain? These are all hallmarks of upper cervical problems.

Now take a pair of shoes that you have worn for more than a short period of time. Observe the soles of the shoes. Are they worn evenly left to right or do they "slant" one way or the other. Shoes should wear evenly front to back and side to side. Sideways slanting wear on your shoes is an indicator that you are not carrying yourself straight.

Finally, have someone observe you as you walk. Do you lean forward or lean to the side as you walk?

All of these symptoms are dead giveaways of an upper cervical spinal issue. However, please note that "passing" these tests doesn't mean you *don't* have an upper cervical problem. But if you do have one or more of these conditions, there's a good chance that you may have a problem.

I am so confident that these are real symptoms that I do my own "diagnosing" when I am in crowds. I notice how people hold themselves and find that it is very easy to pick out the people who have chronic pain issues just by using the head and shoulder "checks." This is the method I use when I refer people to the upper cervical chiropractor, and it works!

As a side note, I find it intriguing that people I encounter with multiple sclerosis (MS) almost always have uneven shoulders. Since MS is a central nervous system disease, I surmise that there could be a connection with the upper cervical spinal problems mentioned previously. More research is necessary in this area.

What finally brought me relief from my alleged fibromyalgia problem was treatment by a National Upper Cervical Chiropractic Association, or NUCCA, chiropractor. Because this treatment was so effective, I am puzzled to this day by the apparent disconnect between mainstream medicine and the obvious relationship between the upper cervical spine and conditions like fibromyalgia.

When I presented my own family doctor with information regarding NUCCA, his eyes sort of glazed over and he slipped the pages I printed for him into a file folder, where they no doubt never saw the light of day again. I never bothered to share this information with the arrogant Doctor Hubris, either, because I knew what his response would be.

I don't believe in the "conspiracy theory" that there are cures being withheld from the public for some nefarious reason. I can only surmise that the reluctance to think outside the box has something to do with the training of mainstream medical personnel. For some reason they cannot accept that there might be a condition that they have not heard of or that they do not know how to treat.

So my advice to you is that you should look past the chemicals that are designed to help you live with the symptoms of fibromyalgia and instead look for their cause. Treat your condition like an injury, not a disease. I personally believe that medical professionals have been looking in the wrong place for the source of fibromyalgia, and that in all likelihood you will find the cause of your pain hidden somewhere in the central nervous system. If that's the case, you should suspect a condition of the upper spine, so have a qualified professional look there first.

In the next chapter, I'll talk about the various alternative medical professionals who can help get to the bottom of your pain. But don't be put off by the term "alternative." As I mentioned earlier, anything outside of the traditional, evidence-based medicine practiced by your family doctor, internist or other physician is considered "alternative." I think you'll find the results of alternative treatment for fibromyalgia will make you a believer in its effectiveness.

CHAPTER 8. Your Pain Relief Team

I'm sure you know there is no shortage of medical doctors who will attempt to manage your fibromyalgia pain. The trick is to find the right one, which as you know I found to be a painful, frustrating experience. As I made the rounds of medical professionals, I had no idea which professional was going to be "the one." It almost became comical—I started labeling every doctor I saw like Borg drones in a "Star Trek" movie. They became "5 of 5," "6 of 6," and so on. It wasn't until I reached "9 of 9" that I started seeing results, until finally, "10 of 10" and "11 of 11" provided my tickets to recovery.

It's really important to understand is that there is no "magic bullet" for fibromyalgia recovery. If your problem, like mine, turns out to be in your spine, it will take a combination of treatments to make an effective recovery. This is the reason that the condition is so difficult to treat—it takes a team of individual professionals, each skilled in different disciplines, to overcome the pain. Case in point: in my search for help I visited two general practitioners (one M.D. and one osteopath), two physical therapists, an eye doctor, a traditional chiropractor, my original NUCCA chiropractor and his successor, two imaging centers, and a massage therapist. So the most important part of putting your pain relief team together is to keep searching until you find the right people.

Having said all this, here is how your team should be comprised:

First, you will need a good, open-minded general practitioner, such as a family practice physician or internist. This may surprise you, considering everything I said about how traditional medical practitioners are fairly clueless about conditions like fibromyalgia. However, your general practitioner is important because you absolutely must rule out the obvious causes of your condition first.

He or she will make sure that the appropriate diagnostics are performed, including X-rays, MRIs, and EKGs (which check the electrical activity in your heart), as well as whatever else can be done to rule out any recognizable causes. He or she is also instrumental in pain management during your treatment and recovery. I say "pain management," not "pain relief," because he or she will only be able to (possibly) take the edge off the pain. You will know you are starting to recover when you start to dial down the prescription pain medication dosages your general practitioner provides. Merely masking the symptoms with drugs and living with your condition is *not* your goal.

Presumably you already have a general practitioner, but if you don't you should find one you like and trust before you proceed any further, and then use him or her to coordinate the efforts between the other professionals you will be using. Do *not* accept the diagnosis that "You have fibromyalgia, here are your medications, have a nice life." If that's the reaction of your physician, find someone new who's open to alternative techniques.

Second, you will need a chiropractor. My condition was an upper cervical muscular/skeletal problem that affected the entire central nervous system. The "skeletal" portion of this problem is addressed by the chiropractor. His or her job is to line up the bones so the pressure is off all of the impinged nerve endings.

As mentioned previously, there are different types of chiropractors, and not all are created equal. My treatment was provided by an upper cervical, or NUCCA, chiropractor. NUCCA chiropractors are specialists who address issues only in the head and neck, something many "traditional" chiropractors won't do. The NUCCA methodology is very gentle and virtually painless, which is a big bonus when even breathing hurts.

There are many different techniques NUCCA chiropractors use on the upper cervical vertebrae, which are known as the atlas and axis, or the C-1 and C-2 vertebrae. To determine how he or she can help, a NUCCA doctor first will take a series of X-rays, among them images of the top bone of the spine (the C-1 or atlas).

If you have an upper cervical problem, the X-ray will show a misalignment in the atlas and the rest of the vertebrae that can be fixed over time by applying gentle, painless pressure. The chiropractor will also use his or her hands to adjust the atlas. There's no twisting or pulling on the body because it only takes slight pressure to realign the spine and relieve nerve pressure. This is accomplished with the activator tool, a small plunger-type device that directs pressure to a specific area of the spine identified by the NUCCA chiropractor.

Traditional chiropractors take a more physical approach to pain relief. They make hands-on adjustments to realign the spine and pelvis and thus take pressure off the nerves. However, if your pain originates in the head or neck, a NUCCA chiropractor may be a better choice.

I give you the benefit of my experience and recommend using a NUCCA chiropractor. I consider my encounter with my two NUCCA chiropractors serendipitous and I hope that God considers this book ample payback for the divine gift He gave me the day I found the advertisement for my NUCCA practitioner in the newspaper. Incidentally, let me reiterate here that I am in no way connected to or compensated by NUCCA for promoting upper cervical treatment in this book. I am only sharing my experiences with you.

Third, you will need a massage therapist. Massage therapy is a crucial part of your recovery. However, you are looking for therapeutic massage, not a gentle, relaxing massage like you'd receive for stress relief. You need a massage therapist who has a true understanding of the head and neck. He or she should be experienced in craniosacral massage (a light-touch head massage) and myofascial release (a type of soft tissue therapy). Combined with treatment by an upper cervical chiropractor, your chances of recovery increase dramatically.

The referral to my massage therapist came from my NUCCA chiropractor, so be sure to ask your own NUCCA chiropractor for a referral to a competent massage therapist. You can also see www.upledger.com for further information on craniosacral massage and a list of practitioners. There is not a specific association for myofascial release therapy, but the internet has a wealth of resources that you can explore.

The reason therapeutic massage works is because when bones are moved out of place, connective tissue forms around them and holds the bones and muscles in the out-of-place position. This places pressure on the nerve endings and presents itself as pain. So although a chiropractor will move the bones into place, the connective tissue will pull them back out of place again.

The massage therapist breaks up the scar tissue that forms on the connective tissue, which allows the bones to stay in the correct position. The massage therapist also can help correctly reposition nerves that have been moved out of place. As an added bonus, the process feels good and relieves much of the pain.

Fourth, you may need a physical therapist. If you have been debilitated for a long period of time, you may need to tone up your muscles, which keeps everything in place even if you are already feeling well. The need for physical therapy depends on your individual situation. Your massage therapist or chiropractor should be able to recommend a good physical therapist if you need one.

Finally, a yoga instructor may help. By taking a yoga class, you will learn a series of postures, or *asanas*, as well as controlled breathing, which will gently help you build core strength and flexibility, both of which can help you overcome pain. Yoga won't provide 100% pain relief, but when combined with NUCCA chiropractic care and therapeutic massage, it really can make you feel better. My NUCCA chiropractor recommends Iyengar yoga, which is a form of Hatha yoga that uses props like blocks, blankets, and straps to support the body so you can safely improve your range of motion.

The first three team members — your general practitioner, chiropractor, and massage therapist — comprise the elements you will need for a successful recovery from fibromyalgia, while the fourth and fifth — the physical therapist and Iyengar yoga teacher — may be needed based on your overall condition. These team members work together and are a natural cure for a painful condition, and should be consulted in the order I've discussed here — otherwise you could find yourself in more pain.

For instance, if you go to a physical therapist before the chiropractor has straightened you out, he or she will succeed in making your situation worse, much like what happened to me. However, both the massage therapist and the physical therapist have much to offer once the chiropractor has been working on you for a while. Use your general practitioner to rule out other causes and for help with controlling pain during the recovery process.

The one downside to this entire process is that you shouldn't expect your insurance to cover all of the expenses for this course of treatment. In my case, my insurance company was happy to pay for all the drugs prescribed to try and relieve my pain, but it was not interested in covering costs associated with fixing my condition. But the relief I finally found made the out-of-pocket expenses well worth the cost.

It's also important to remember that this process takes time, and you must truly be patient on the road to a total recovery. It may take months or even years to achieve a complete recovery. But just remember: your condition can take decades to develop, so it only makes sense that it takes some time to unravel. The recovery process can be compared to peeling an onion, one layer at a time. The good news is that the gradual improvement during the treatment process is very encouraging and your spirit will soar as you improve!

I've included a list of resources for the alternative techniques I've mentioned here at the end of this book, as well as a list of NUCCA practitioners.

CHAPTER 9. Recovery Time

For those who have visited a NUCCA practitioner and found a problem with their atlas their next question is always "How quickly do I recover." It is important to note that the NUCCA method is not a magic cure or elixir. It is a natural healing process. The chiropractor does not heal the injury; he is simply putting the body in a position to heal itself. For this reason the recovery is a slow methodical process.

On the plus side there is no surgery or drugs involved in this rehabilitation process. You need only stick with the program and see it through to the end to obtain relief.

While you may obtain some pain relief on your first visit, more than likely your progress will be in small incremental steps over a period of time. In my case the healing was gradual over a five-year period. Keep in mind that I was completely debilitated before treatment started — essentially I was almost immobilized and ready to be fitted for a wheel chair. After just a few months I was moving around again and starting to return to a "normal" life.

Every injury to the atlas is different and therefore every recovery is different as well. The atlas displacement will vary depending on the angle of misalignment as well as the movement that has occurred. These variables will effect what areas of the body are affected by the injury and the subsequent healing.

The healing process is best described as the "peeling of an onion." Just like removing the layers of an onion, the most recent symptoms will start to fade first followed by the earlier symptoms until the very first symptom is the last to fade.

Progress may seem to be haphazard. It is not unusual to feel tired and worn out the day after an atlas adjustment but then to feel significantly better several days later. This is "normal" for the healing process and should be seen as a good sign.

You can take action to improve your comfort during the healing process. Applying ice immediately after an adjustment will reduce inflammation. Taking anti-inflammatory medications (such as Motrin, Advil, or Aspirin) can also help. Consult your General Practitioner for help in this area. Nerves have already been irritated by the misalignment of the atlas so as the NUCCA practitioner works around the atlas these nerves will become further irritated as a result. This added inflammation will cause pain after adjustments so anything you can do to reduce it will help with the pain. You will find as you recover you require less and less medication to control pain. This is a good way to track the slow recovery process.

Much like the condition itself, the recovery can result in some strange and unusual symptoms some of which I would like to mention here.

When the body is twisted off center and the head is tilted your brain makes an adjustment. You can see this for yourself by standing in front of a mirror and closing your eyes. Move your head left, right, up, and down. After you have done that while keeping your eyes closed straighten your head.

Most patients with atlas displacement will open their eyes and find that even though they thought that their head was level it was actually tilted to one side or the other. This is because in order to keep your balance the brain has adjusted to the angled head.

This occurs automatically for you and is not a problem until the chiropractor starts to straighten your body back out. As the body straightens the head incrementally levels back out. Unfortunately though the brain will now perceive this as being "out of balance" since it has become accustomed to having the head held at an angle.

The brain will automatically correct itself over a period of time. The problem is that while the brain is adjusting to the head being straight you will feel dizzy. You may stagger when walking and have trouble staying upright. The sensation is the same as getting off of a boat after being on the water all day. As disturbing as this is, this is a normal recovery progression.

Your sense of smell and taste may also be affected. This is because these nerves are near the atlas. As recovery occurs you may find that your sense of taste changes. Foods that were appealing to you are no longer. You may find that you appreciate other foods more.

As pressure is removed from nerves you may get "shooting pains" in different areas of the body. This is akin to the feelings you get when a rubber band is tied around a finger and then removed. While these pains can be disturbing what is actually occurring is the nerve endings are coming back to life, another good sign.

I found that after an adjustment I would feel fatigue. It was not unusual to go home and fall asleep. The amount of sleep needed will lesson as time goes by so it can also be an indicator of improvement.

Perhaps the most important components of your recovery are psychological. Typical atlas injuries degenerate over a long period of time and many sufferers have experienced a slow debilitating decline before they find qualified help. As a result both hope and patience are key components of your recovery.

Patience is critical because the recovery process is slow. The general rule is to allow one month of recovery time for every year that has lapsed since the initial injury. In many cases you may not be aware of the initial injury so the time will be difficult to determine. In any event, the recovery time always varies by individual so it is impossible to quantify exactly how long it will take. Therefore, be patient!

Hand in hand with patience is hope. This can be a great morale boost for those who have suffered a long time. I found that in my case even though the recovery was slow just knowing that a recovery was in process gave me extra enthusiasm for the journey.

This is important because it will get you through the process. When I started my atlas adjustments I was receiving two per week. Eventually I went down to less than one per month. It was the hope that I finally could recover that enabled me to take the time and effort to see the treatment through to recovery. I hope that you find that this encouragement enables you to persevere as well.

CHAPTER 10. A Brighter Future

I have shared with you a painful chapter in my life. I am compelled to do so because of the many people I have encountered with similar circumstances. These people all have one thing in common — they have fallen through the cracks in the traditional medical system into a dark hole of pain and anguish from which there appears to be no escape. As I have encountered these people I have been compelled to share this information in order to help the human condition, in order to relieve their pain and anguish in any way that I might.

I have seen veritable miracles performed in the upper cervical chiropractor's office. Aside from my own case, I have seen a woman who could not walk become pain-free. A child who could not talk became able to speak. I saw a woman who could not stand on her own gleefully prance about. Upper cervical care can do all this and more. There is no doubt in my mind that injury to the upper spine is the most misunderstood and misdiagnosed injury to the body.

In some cases a car accident or similar jolt to the spine can cause the injury. Other mundane causes can be poor posture, injury at birth, awkwardly stepping off a curb — or going out for a bucket of chicken.

Regardless of the cause, the symptoms of this injury are many and cruel. The central nervous system screams out vengeance for injuries against it in the form of pain, suffering, numbness, fatigue, and any number of other debilitating symptoms. Since the symptoms are so random, the cause is difficult to pinpoint. But a few simple X-rays can verify if your issues are caused by upper cervical injury or misalignment.

In my case, I surmise that it was the handling of my original injury (that awkward exit from a car, coupled with a step down onto a manhole cover) that caused my condition. When the C-6 vertebra in my spine shifted out of place the tension holding the spinal discs in place was reduced. This caused all of the discs to shift, and when my neck was rotated by my doctor the nerves became tangled between the discs all along the spine. The physical therapy then aggravated the nerves and caused the pain. I would never have recovered from this condition without the manipulation of the upper cervical spine and correct repositioning of the nerves done by my NUCCA chiropractor.

Fibromyalgia cost me five years of my life. To recover I had to overcome a myriad of obstacles. I encountered physicians who did not believe I was injured, and diagnostic tools that did not reveal a problem. The medical system was not prepared to deal with my injury. I discovered I had what I refer to as "coverless" insurance: While I made payments every month the insurance company failed to cover my condition. I paid for all of the treatment that helped me recover out of my own pocket. Apparently, the insurance industry doesn't understand this injury, either.

I have come a long way since October 2006. As of July 2012, I have my life back. I do the things I want to do, and I am working on building my strength back up by taking long walks as often as I can. Had I settled for the initial diagnosis I would probably still be in debilitating pain.

On the day I met Dr. Rich and started toward my recovery, I could feel my soul lighten. Hopelessness is a terrible thing that can be just as debilitating as any disease or condition can be. I sincerely pray that I have extended hope to you, that there is a way you can recover and that your future can be bright again. Assemble your team, and don't settle for practitioners who aren't sympathetic and helpful. Find the strength to persevere.

May God bless you and be with you every step of the way.

RESOURCES

American Massage Therapy Association
500 Davis Street, Suite 900
Evanston, IL 60201-4695
Toll-free (877) 905-0577
Phone: (847) 864-0123
Fax: (847) 864-5196
Website: www.amatamassage.org
Email: info@amtamassage.org

Centers for Disease Control and Prevention
www.cdc.gov

Iyengar Yoga Association of the United States
1952 First Avenue South, Suite 1B
Seattle, WA, 98134
Phone: (206) 623-3562
Website: http://iynaus.org
Email: iynaus@iynaus.org

National Fibromyalgia Association
2121 S. Towne Centre Place, Suite 300
Anaheim, CA 92806
Phone: (714) 921-0150
Fax: (714) 921-6920
Website: www.fmaware.org

National Upper Cervical Chiropractic Association
1500 Sunday Drive, Suite 102
Raleigh, NC 27609
Toll-free (800) 541-5799
Office (919) 573-5443
Fax (877) 558-0410
Website: www.nucca.org

Email: infor@nucca.org

GLOSSARY

Atlas: The first cervical (neck) vertebra, which supports the head. Also known as C-1.

Chiropractic adjustment: A manipulation of bones by chiropractic professional.

Connective tissue: The body tissue between your muscles and nerves.

Craniosacral massage: A type of gentle healing massage that enhances the functioning of the craniosacral system, which includes the cranium and spine. Its purpose is to bring pain relief, among other benefits.

Evidence-based medicine: Medical practices based on evidence gained from scientific research and proven clinical practices.

Fibromyalgia: A painful chronic condition of the nervous system that results in musculoskeletal pain and fatigue.

Massage therapist: A person who manually manipulates the soft tissues of the body for pain relief and tissue healing, among other benefits.

Myofascial release: A type of hands-on bodywork that releases tension in the connective tissue of the body.

National Upper Cervical Chiropractor Association: Organization devoted to the healing processes possible through upper cervical care.

NUCCA: Acronym for National Upper Cervical Chiropractor Association.

Physical therapy: Treatment of a condition using techniques that exercise and stretch the muscles.

Spinal subluxation: A medical term that refers to a misalignment of the spine that occurs when one or more vertebrae are out of alignment with the others, causing pain and a host of other symptoms.

Therapeutic massage: Massage of the soft tissues of the body to prevent and alleviate pain and promote health and wellness.

Traditional medicine: The generally-accepted medical practices that may or may not help with your fibromyalgia.

Upper cervical: Refers to the top two vertebrae of the spine (the atlas and axis, also known as C-1 and C-2).

Upper cervical chiropractor: A chiropractor who specializes in misalignments of the top two bones of the spine (the atlas and axis) to restore health and eliminate pain.

Vertebrae: The round discs that comprise the spinal column.

APPENDIX A. NUCCA
PRACTITIONERS USA

(Arranged by U.S. State)

Dr. Anthony Rumsey
Rumsey Spinal Care
8301 Briarwood St.
Ste. 103
Anchorage, AK 99815
Phone: (907) 336-0200
Fax: (907) 336-0201
http://www.rumseyspinalcare.com

Dr. Gerald Martin
840 W. University Dr.
Ste. 7
Mesa, AZ 85201
Phone: 480-964-1129
Fax: 480-649-4375
Email: drgemartin@yahoo.com

Dr. G. Miguel Gracey
Gracey Clinic
1530 N. Country Club Drive
#18
Mesa, AZ 85201
Phone: 480-964-4407
Fax: 480-964-8550
Email: graceychiropractic@gracey.phxcoxmail.com

Dr. Abigail Longner

Longner Chiropractic
3712 Hwy 95
Ste B
Bullhead City, AZ 86442
Phone: 928-763-9333
Email: chiroabi@gmail.com

Dr. Jack Wheatley
840 West University Drive
#7
Mesa, AZ 85201
Phone: 480-964-1129
Fax: 480-649-4375
Email: jgus44@cox.net

Dr. Glenn Cripe
Cripe Upper Cervical Center
1501 Westcliff Dr.
Suite 210
Newport Beach, CA 92660
Phone: 949-631-5171
Fax: 949-631-6992
Email: glenn@cripe-nucca.com
http://www.cripeuppercervicalcenter.com

Dr. Steven MacDonald
718 Lighthouse Ave
Suite A
Pacific Grove, CA 93950
Phone: 831-375-9528
Fax: 831-375-9529
Email: drmacnucca1@sbcglobal.net
http://www.drmacnucca.com

Dr. Michael Zabelin

Cow Hollow Chiropractic
3014 Fillmore St
2nd Floor
San Francisco, CA 94123
Phone: 415-931-5000
Fax: 415-931-5080
Email: drzabelin@gmail.com

Dr. Shannon Connor
1617 Westcliff Drive
Suite 210
Newport Beach, CA 92660
Phone: 949-642-5660
Fax: 949-642-5660
Email: drshannonconnor@att.net
http://www.drshannonconnor.com

Dr. Steven Danaher
Precision Chiropractic
712 D Street
Suite J
San Rafael, CA 94901
Phone: 415 457-9600
Email: StevenDanaher@hotmail.com
http://www.marinnucca.com

Dr. Kathy Doyle
400 40th Street
Suite C
Oakland, CA 94609
Phone: 510-601-6325
Email: drdoyle@ymail.com

Dr. Donald Erwin

Erwin Spinal Care
900 Fulton Ave.
Ste 102
Sacramento, CA 95825-4516
Phone: 916-973-0623
Fax: 916-973-0338
Email: uppercdc@sbcglobal.net

Dr. Tymothy Flory
Atlas Spinal Care
2335 W Foothill Blvd, Suite 20
Upland, CA 91786
Phone: 909 982-9100
Fax: 909 257-3990
Email: DrFlory@me.com
http://www.AtlasSpinalCare.com

Dr. Brett Gottlieb
Gottlieb Chiropractic & Health Services, Inc.
4401 Hazel Avenue
Suite 100
Fair Oaks, CA 95628
Phone: 916-965-7155
Fax: 916-966-6085
Email: drgnuc@earthlink.net
http://www.painfreelife.net

Dr. Armen Manoucherian
Cripe Upper Cervical Center
1501 Westcliff Drive Suite 210
Newport Beach, CA 92660
Phone: 949-631-5171
Fax: 949-631-6992
Email: manoucherian@gmail.com

Dr. Jack Manuele

Jack D. Manuele, DC
1930 W. Glenoaks Blvd
Suite 4
Glendale, CA 91201
Phone: 818-842-4444
Fax: 818-842-4444
Email: jmanueledc@att.net

Dr. Christina Meakim
San Francisco Family Spinal Care
505 Beach St
Ste 110
San Francisco, CA 94133
Phone: 415-771-7071
Fax: 415-771-7073
Email: drmeakim@sffamilyspinalcare.com
http://www.sffamilyspinalcare.com

Dr. Stephen Nakano
1808 West 152nd Street
Gardena, CA 90249
Phone: 310-323-3370
Fax: 310-323-0233
Email: snakanodc@yahoo.com

 Dr. Jamie Stern
Sunnyvale Family Chiropractic
130 South Frances Street
Sunnyvale, CA 94086
Phone: 415-308-7636
Email: Jamie_stern@ yahoo.com

Dr. Pete Tsiglieris

Advanced Spinal Care
643 Bair Island Road, Suite 208
Redwood City, CA 94063
Phone: 650-595-0500
Email: drtsiglieris@yahoo.com
http://www.BayAreaNuccaCare.com

Dr. Brian Cripe
Cripe Upper Cervical Center
1501 Westcliff Dr.
Ste. 210
Newport Beach, CA 92660
Phone: 949-631-5171
Fax: 949-631-6992
Email: drbrian@cripeuppercervicalcenter.com
http://www.cripeuppercervicalcenter.com

Dr. Bill Davis
Breath of Life Chiropractic
161 Thunder Drive
Suite 104
Vista, CA 92083
Phone: 760-945-1345
Fax: 760-945-1377
Email: nuccadoctordavis@yahoo.com
http://www.nuccawellness.com

Dr. Jamie Kaszer
Back Into Balance
462 Stevens Ave.
Ste 306
Solana Beach, CA 92075
Phone: 858-847-3333
Fax: 858-847-3334
Email: info@whatisnucca.com
http://www.WhatIsNUCCA.com

Dr. Giancarlo Licata
Licata Chiropractic, Inc.
125 Wheeler Avenue
Suite A
Arcadia, CA 91006
Phone: 626-446-3400
Fax: 626-446-3404
Email: licataclinic@gmail.com
http://www.licataclinic.com

Dr. Andrea Pritchett
Vital Life Wellness Center
7451 Village Parkway
Dublin, CA 94568
Phone: 925-829-7900
Fax: 925-369-7191
Email: nucca@vlifewellness.com
http://www.vlifewellness.com

Dr. Rebecca Basilio
Breath of Life
161 Thunder Dr Suite 104
Vista, CA 92083
Phone: 760-945-1345
Fax: 760-945-1377
Email: drbecca@nuccawellness.com
http://www.nuccawellness.com

Dr. Robert Basilio

Breath of Life
161 Thunder Dr.
Vista, CA 92083
Phone: 760-945-1345
Fax: 760-945-1377
Email: drrob@nuccawellness.com
http://www.nuccawellness.com

Dr. Julia Ciano
Dr. Julia Ciano
451 Parkfair Drive Suite 4
Sacramento, CA 95864
Phone: 916-484-6882
Fax: 916-484-7078
Email: drjuliaciano@yahoo.com
http://www.drciano.com

Dr. Nathaniel Elkins
11500 W. Olympic Blvd
Ste. 364
Los Angeles, CA 90064
Phone: 310-445-8300
Fax: 310-933-4679
Email: drelkinschiropractic@gmail.com
http://www.nuccala.com

Dr. Wendy Lanser
Lanser Chiropractic Inc.
990 W. Fremont Ave
Ste P
Sunnyvale, CA 94087
Phone: 408-245-5454
Fax: 408-245-5656
Email: drlanser@lanserchiropractic.com
http://www.lanserchiropractic.com

Dr. James Pietrek
Pietrek Spinal Care
16959 Bernardo Center Drive
Suite 215
San Diego, CA 92128
Phone: 858-676-1218
Fax: 858-676-5316
Email: drpietrek@pietrekspinalcare.com
http://www.pietrekspinalcare.com

Dr. Kenny Sheppard
Sheppard Spine and Sports
634 Stevens Ave.
Solana Beach, CA 92075
Phone: 858-350-6290
Fax: 858-350-6775
Email: drkennysheppard@yahoo.com
http://www.Sheppardspineandsports.com

Dr. Dan Spinato
9320 Carmel Mountain Road
Suite B
San Diego, CA 92129
Phone: 858-484-0444
Fax: 858-484-0552
Email: dan.spinato@yahoo.com
http://danspinato.com

Dr. Alex Tam

Absolute Family Chiropractic
1490 Alamo Dr. Suite B
Vacaville, CA 95687
Phone: 707-474-5688
Fax: 707-474-5658
Email: drtam@AbsoluteFamilyChiropractic.com
http://www.AbsoluteFamilyChiropractic.com

Dr. Surachna Virdi-Hulsebus
Cow Hollow Chiropratic
3014 Fillmore St.
2nd Floor
San Francisco, CA 94123
Email: dr.svirdidc@gmail.com

Dr. James Weiss
Atlas Spinal Care
2335 W Foothill Blvd
Ste 20
Upland, CA 91786
Phone: 909-982-9100
Fax: 909-257-3990
Email: atlasspinalcare@gmail.com
http://www.atlasspinalcare.com

Dr. Chris Woolf
Woolf Spinal Care
391 Taylor Boulevard
Suite 130
Pleasant Hill, CA 94523
Phone: (925) 798-1770
Fax: (925) 798-1770
Email: drwoolf@woolfspinalcare.com
http://woolfspinalcare.com

Dr. Thomas Groover

Groover Clinic
2725 Iris Avenue
Boulder, CO 80304
Phone: 303-442-7772
Fax: 303-442-2426
Email: drgroover@comcast.net
http://www.grooverclinic.com

Dr. David Jung
Jung Spinal Care
7600 E. Arapahoe Rd
Suite 106
Centennial, CO 80112
Phone: 720-489-6040
Fax: 720-489-6063
Email: david@nuccadenver.com

Dr. Mario Chavez
Vita Nova Spinal Care
5437 S Prince St.
Littleton, CO 80120
Phone: (303) 798-8672 (VNSC)
Email: drchavez@vitanovaspinalcare.com
http://www.VitaNovaSpinalCare.com

Dr. Scott Gamm
Balance Wellness and Chiropractic Center
415 W Rockrimmon Blvd
Ste 400
Colorado Springs, CO 80919
Phone: 719-265-0115
Fax: 719-265-0116
Email: dr.scottgamm@yahoo.com
http://www.balancecolorado.com

Dr. Deana Burd

Spinal Specialists of Delaware
300 Christiana Medical Center
Newark, DE 19702
Phone: 302-731-0869
Fax: 302-292-0669
Email: doctorburd@verizon.net
http://www.spinalspecialistsofdelaware.com

Dr. John Dunn
NUCCA Board Certified
Dunn Chiropractic
1213 North Monroe St
Tallahassee, FL 32303
Phone: 850-222-1171
Fax: 850-222-1174
Email: dunnet@talstar.com

Dr. Justin Brown
Friends & Family Spinal Care
4674 Coral Ridge Drive
Coral Springs, FL 33076
Phone: 954-369-1212
Fax: 954-757-2009
Email: drbrown@familyspinalcare.com
http://www.familyspinalcare.com

Dr. Jeanie Froman-Bohall
Chiropractic Discovery & Wellness
9191 RG Skinner Pky
Suite 503
Jacksonville, FL 32256
Phone: 904-738-8189
Fax: 904-212-1612
Email: froman75@yahoo.com
http://www.chirodiscoveryjax.com

Dr. Michael Thomas
Thomas Chiropractic Care
10252 S. US Hwy 441
Ste 1
Belleview, FL 34420
Phone: 352-245-6169
Fax: 352-347-0748
Email: nuccadc@earthlink.net
http://www.uppercervicaldr.com

Dr. Gregory Gumberich
Gumberich Family Chiropractic
6426 Lake Worth Road
Lake Worth, FL 33463
Phone: 561-964-1600
Fax: 561-964-5404
Email: ggumberich@yahoo.com
http://www.jogchiro.com

Dr. Jason Nitzsche
Orlando Spine Center
1009 Webster Ave
Orlando, FL 32804
Phone: 407-578-2225
Fax: 407-253-4335
Email: info@gentlespinecare.com
http://www.gentlespinecare.com

Dr. Bryan Salminen

Alpha Spine Center
12220 Birmingham Hwy
Suite 40
Milton, GA 30004
Phone: 770-777-2377
Fax: 770-777-2527
Email: info@alphaspinecenter.com
http://www.alphaspinecenter.com

Dr. Yoshiro Yajima
Izumi Chiropractic
5000 Winter Chapel Rd.
Suite 1
Dorabille, GA 30360
Phone: 678-855-6611
Fax: 678-528-5097
Email: holistichealthsolutions@hotmail.com

Dr. Joseph Breuwet
Upper Cervical Hawaii
1600 Kapiolani Blvd.
Suite 1421
Honolulu, HI 96814
Phone: 808-638-1313
Fax: 808-942-9493
Email: uppercervicalhawaii@hawaii.rr.com
http://www.uppercervicalhawaii.com

Dr. Kelly Mix-Stork
Stork Spinal Care
1961 N. Locust Grove Road
Meridian, ID 83646
Phone: 208-888-8797
Fax: 208-888-8797
Email: drmixstork@yahoo.com
http://www.storkspinalcare.com

Dr. Trever Neville
Neville Spinal Balance
2145 West Broadway St
Idaho Falls, ID 83402
Phone: 208-522-3130
Fax: 208-522-3168
Email: spinalbalance1@gmail.com

Dr. Robert Stork
Stork Spinal Care P.C.
1961 N. Locust Grove Road
Meridian, ID 83646
Phone: 208-888-8797
Fax: 208-888-8799
Email: robertstorkdc@yahoo.com
http://www.storkspinalcare.com

Dr. Marshall Dickholtz, Jr.
Healthsmart
2565 Shermer Road
Northbrook, IL 60062
Phone: 847-272-1000
Fax: 847-272-9742
Email: healthsmart1@sbcglobal.net
http://www.NUCCACARE.COM

Dr. Marshall Dickholtz, Sr.
Chiropractic Offices
3420 West Peterson Ave
Chicago, IL 60659
Phone: 773-267-0020
Fax: 773-267-6004
Email: dmarshallsr@gmail.com
http://www.nuccadickholtzsr.com

Dr. Jeremy Barone
Barone Spinal Care
937 N. Plum Grove Rd., Ste. B
Schaumburg, IL 60173
Phone: 847-619-7579
Fax: 847-619-6845
Email: JBarone@BaroneSpinalCare.com
http://www.baronespinalcare.com

Dr. Nathalie Bloom
Nucare
3330 Dundee Road
Suite C-8
Northbrook, IL 60062
Phone: 847-480-1718
Fax: 847-480-1925
Email: nucare@netzero.com
http://www.atnucare.com

Dr. Tom Bryant
Health Solutions Precision Spinal Care LLC
105 Revere Dr.
Suite F-1
Northbrook, IL 60062
Phone: 224-723-5728
Fax: 224-723-5726
Email: drbryantnucca@msn.com

Dr. Young Chung
NUCCA Wellness Clinic of Chicago
3420 W. Peterson Ave.
Chicago, IL 60659
Phone: 773-267-0020
Fax: 773-267-6004
Email: ChungDC@gmail.com
http://www.nuccawcc.com

Dr. Daniel Fedeli
The Balancing Center
1165 N Clark St
Suite 602
Chicago, IL 60610
Phone: 312-787-7222
Fax: 312-787-7227
Email: drdan@thebalancingcenter.com
http://www.TheBalancingCenter.com

Dr. Bruce Giffen
Giffen Spinal Care, Ltd.
600 First Bank Dr.
Ste B
Palatine, IL 60067
Phone: 847-963-9697
Fax: 847-963-9695
Email: bpgiffen@juno.com
http://www.nuccadrgiffen.com

Dr. Daiki Ishiyama
HealthSmart
2565 Shermer Rd.
Northbrook, IL 60062
Phone: 847-272-1000
Fax: 847-272-9472
Email: daiki.dc@gmail.com
http://www.nuccacare.com/

Dr. Caroline Bergeron

Health Solutions Comprehensive Quality Care LLC
5550 W. Touhy Ave.
Ste 202
Skokie, IL 60077
Phone: 847-329-7501
Fax: 847-329-7507
Email: health.solutions.cqc@gmail.com
http://www.healthsolutionscqc.com

Dr. Philip Schalow
1st Step Chiropractic SC
4519 Highcrest Rd
Rockford, IL 61107
Phone: 815-398-4500
Fax: 815-398-4515
Email: pkschalow@hotmail.com
http://www.myrockfordchiropractor.com

Dr. Valeri Briski
1st Place Chiropractic
1750 E Main St. Suite 140
St. Charles, IL 60174
Phone: 630-584-5200
Fax: 630-584-8370
Email: vjbriski@gmail.com
http://www.1stplacechiropractic.com

Dr. Kyrie Kleinfelter
1st Place Chiropractic
1750 E. Main St.
Ste 140
St. Charles, IL 60174
Phone: 630-584-5200
Fax: 630-584-8370
Email: drkleinfelter@yahoo.com
http://www.1stPlaceChiropractic.com

Dr. Bryan Laneville
880 75th St.
Willowbrook, IL 60527
Phone: 630-325-5522
Fax: 630-325-5535
Email: info@chicagolandnucca.com
http://www.chicagolandnucca.com

Dr. Erich Griffith
Uptown Chiropractic Clinic
827 S. Union St.
Ste 210
Warsaw, IN 46580
Phone: 574-269-7726
Fax: 574-269-7728 call bef
Email: dregrif@gmail.com

Dr. Barbara Read
Read Health Center, Inc.
1606 Golden Aspen Dr.
Ste 101
Ames, IA 50010
Phone: 515-233-8880
Fax: 515-233-8882
Email: bkreaddc@hotmail.com
http://DrBarbaraRead.com
 Dr. Deb Sesker
Balance First Chiropractic Center, PC
974 73rd Street
Suite 27
Des Moines, IA 50324
Phone: 515-267-8851
Fax: 515-267-8894
Email: balancefirst@gmail.com
http://www.chiropracticdsm.com

Dr. Robert Gilbert
Dr. Robert J Gilbert DC
901 E Kimberly Rd
Suite 17
Davenport, IA 52807
Phone: 563-322-5739
Fax: 563-884-4232
Email: gilbertrdc@aol.com

Dr. Lance Kellow
Authentic Spinal Care, PLC
2900 100th St.
Suite 204
Urbandale, IA 50322
Phone: 515-270-1700

Dr. David Chalke
Chalke Chiropractic
412 Adams Street
Paducah, KY 42001
Phone: 270-442-3988
Fax: 270-442-4645
Email: drchalke@gmail.com
http://drchalke.com

Fax: 515-270-1744
Email: authenticspinalcare@live.com
http://www.authenticspinalcare.com

Dr. Chris Faler

Premier Chiropractic
1120 N. Cause Blvd.
Suite 2
Mandeville, LA 70471
Phone: 985-674-5855
Fax: 985-674-5854
Email: drfaler@aol.com
http://www.drfaler.com

Dr. Andrew Smyth
106 Access Road
Unit #7
Norwood, MA 02062
Phone: 781-255-5565
Fax: 781-255-5564
Email: drsmyth@nespinalcare.com
http://www.nespinalcare.com

Dr. Richard Cicala
Balanced Living Chiropractic
441 S. Livernois Road Suite 265
Rochester Hlls, Michigan 48307
Phone: 248-652-7225
www.balancedlivingchiropracticplc.com

Dr. Kerry Johnson
Johnson Spinal Care Associates PA
14859 Energy Way
Apple Valley, MN 55124
Phone: 952-432-3333
Fax: 952-432-4444
Email: kerry@johnsonspinalcare.com
http://www.johnsonspinalcare.com

Dr. Jeffrey Leach

Living Well Chiropractic, P.C.
3140 Harbor Lane N
Ste. 102
Plymouth, MN 55447
Phone: 763-230-7333
Fax: 763-230-7335
Email: drjeff@livingwellmn.com
http://www.livingwellmn.com

Dr. Rodd Bruntjen
Mighty Oak Chiropractic
2233 Energy Park Drive
Ste 500
Saint Paul, MN 55108
Phone: 651-646-2233
Fax: 651-646-2936
Email: nucca2@mightyoak.org
http://www.mightyoak.org

Dr. Todd Sands
Precision Chiropractic Center
119 S.W. 6th St.
Ste 100
Rochester, MN 55902
Phone: 507-287-6041
Fax: 507-287-6438
Email: drtmsands@yahoo.com
http://www.precisionchiropracticcenter.net

Dr. Matthew Flory

Delta Spinal Care
8403 Maryland Avenue
Clayton, MO 63105
Phone: 877-725-3358
Fax: 314-725-1733
Email: drmatt@deltaspinalcare.com

Dr. Chris Maffit
Delta Spinal Care
8403 Maryland Ave
Clayton, MO 63015
Phone: 877-725-3358
Fax: 314-725-1733
Email: drchris@deltaspinalcare.com

Dr. Chris Wambeke
Flip Spinal Care
301 E. 2nd St.
Ste.1D P. O. Box 2039
Whitefish, MT 59937
Phone: 406-862-3547
Fax: 406-862-7895
Email: flipchiropractic@yahoo.com
http://flipspinalcare.com

Dr. Drew Drummond
5332 S. 138th St.
Ste. 210
Omaha, NE 68137
Phone: 402-452-3400
Fax: 402-452-3401
Email: spinalbalance@yahoo.com
http://spinalbalancehc.com

Dr. Marcella Ziska

Body in Harmony Chiropractic Center
11850 Nicholas Street
Suite 220
Omaha, NE 68132
Phone: (402) 614-4201
Fax: (402) 614-4520
Email: drz@bodyinharmonyomaha.com
http://www.bodyinharmonyomaha.com

Dr. Allen Huff
Precision Spinal Care
620 S. Jeffers St.
North Platte, NE 69101
Phone: 308-221-2880
Email: allen@nucca.info
http://www.nucca.info

Dr. Dennis Salisbury
Salisbury Chiropractic Clinic
1015 W. 8th St.
Chadron, NE 69337
Phone: 308-432-2015
Fax: 308-432-3975
Email: drdsalis@hotmail.com

Dr. Matt Wehr
Precision Spinal Care
620 S. Jeffers St
North Palatte, NE 69101
Phone: 308-221-2880
Email: matt@nucca.info
http://www.nucca.info

Dr. Robert Goodman

Nevada Spine Institute
1485 W. Warm Springs Road
Suite 103-A
Henderson, NV 89014
Phone: 702-450-0990
Fax: 702-450-0993
Email: drgoodman@nvspine.com
http://www.nvspine.com

Dr. Devin Luzod
Spinal Care of Nevada
8910 W Tropicana
Ste 6
Las Vegas, NV 89147
Phone: 702-944-4673
Fax: 702-944-4672
Email: DrD@DrDevin.com
http://www.DrDevin.com

Dr. Thor Mongie
Renaissance Health Centre
2820 W Charleston Blvd
Ste A6
Las Vegas, NV 89102
Phone: 702-258-7860
Fax: 702-258-5487
Email: thormongie@hotmail.com
http://www.iwholeheath.com

Dr. Sarah Johnson

Spine Wellness Center
3085 East Russell Road
Suite E
Las Vegas, NV 89120
Phone: 702-433-8333
Fax: 702-433-4632
Email: drjohnson@spinewellnesscenter.com
http://www.spinewellnesscenter.com

Dr. James LeFever
Summerlin Chiropractic Associates
1215 S. Fort Apache Rd.
Ste. 140
Las Vegas, NV 89117
Phone: (702) 362-0336
Fax: (702) 362-9680
Email: drlefever@yahoo.com
http://www.LasVegasNUCCAChiropractor.com

Dr. Christopher Dawson
Quest Spinal Health Center
600 State Street
Suite A
Portsmouth, NH 03801
Phone: 603-427-1100
Fax: 603-427-5595
Email: quest4health@mac.com
http://www.quest4wellness.com

Dr. Larry Arbeitman

Upper Cervical Chiropractic of Monmouth, LLC
25 Kilmer Drive
Building 3 #101
Morganville, NJ 07751
Phone: 732-617-9355
Fax: 732-617-9334
Email: nuccadr@uccofmonmouth.com
http://www.uccofmonmouth.com

Dr. Lonnie Pond
NUCCA Board Certified
Pond Chiropractic Health Center PA
2600 Farmington Ave., Ste. A
PO Box 2332
Farmington, NM 87499
Phone: 505-325-5992
Fax: 505-327-5741
Email: pondchiropractic@msn.com

Dr. Irene Adamczuk
1031 Titus Ave
Rochester, NY 14617
Phone: 585-342-7707
Email: irkac1@frontiernet.net

Dr. Alison Bramer-Cummings
Inner Balance Chiropractic
2800 Sweet Home Rd
Ste 1
Amherst, NY 14228
Phone: (716) 210-1060
Fax: (716) 210-1077
Email: dralison@innerbalancechiro.com
http://www.innerbalancechiro.com

Dr. Michael D'Avanzo

Liberty Wellness and Chiropractic
232 East 66th St.
New York, NY 10065
Phone: 212-785-9620
Fax: 212-935-7278
Email: drdavanzo@lwcmanhattan.com
http://www.lwcmanhattan.com

Dr. George Gertner
Upper Cervical Chiropractic of New York, PC
20 Old Mamaroneck Road
Ste 1C
White Plains, NY 10605
Phone: 914-686-6200
Fax: 914-686-6237
Email: drgertner@ucc-ny.com
http://www.ucc-ny.com

Dr. Michael Polsinelli
Advanced Spinal Care Center
27970 Chardon Rd
Willoughby Hills, OH 44092
Phone: 440-943-6411
Fax: 440-943-6716
Email: drp@spinalalignment.com
http://www.spinalalignment.com

Dr. Geoffrey Besso
Besso Clinic Of Chiropractic Inc.
2071 Graham Road
Stow, OH 44224
Phone: 330-689-1234
Fax: 330-689-1235
Email: drgbesso@gmail.com
http://www.bessoclinic.com

Dr. Gregory Goffe
Goffe Chiropractic Center
387 Regency Ridge Dr.
Dayton, OH 45459
Phone: 937-435-1895
Fax: 937-435-1884
Email: drgoffe@drgoffe.com
http://www.drgoffe.com

Dr. James Terry McCoskey
Living Well Spine Center
1145 Channingway Drive
Fairborn, OH 45324
Phone: 937-878-1071
Fax: 937-878-2616
Email: NUCCA1st@aol.com
http://www.livingwellspinecenter.com

Dr. Douglas Paul
Nu-Chiropractic, Inc.
1335 Dublin Rd., Ste. 75-A
Columbus, OH 43215
Phone: 614-485-9320
Fax: 614-485-9321
Email: drdjpaul1@aol.com
http://nu-chiropractic.com

Dr. Danielle Rice
Worthington Family Chiropractic
57 E. Wilson Bridge Rd.
Ste 200
Worthington, OH 43085
Phone: 614-785-9999
Fax: 614-785-9995
Email: drdaniellerice@yahoo.com
http://www.drdaniellerice.com

Dr. Steven Risner
Risner Spinal Center
1640 Tiffin Ave.
Ste B
Findlay, OH 45840
Phone: 419-422-7677
Fax: 419-422-7673
Email: ohiosnuccadoc@hotmail.com
http://risnerspinalcenter.com

Dr. Robert Brooks
Brooks Spinal Care
1722 South Carson
Suite 3100
Tulsa, OK 74119-4643
Phone: 918-587-7111
Fax: 918-587-1177
Email: healing@brooksspinalcare.com
http://www.brooksspinalcare.com

Dr. Conrad Trapp
Trapp Spinal Care
2017 S. Elm Place
Suite 100
Broken Arrow, OK 74012
Phone: 918-449-9555
Fax: 918-449-9559
Email: ctrappdc@hotmail.com
http://www.trappspinalcare.com

Dr. Nick Bagnaro

Health and Stability Spinal Care
10020-A South Mingo Rd
Tulsa, OK 74133
Phone: 918-991-5427
Fax: 877-335-6779
Email: drbagnaro@gmail.com
http://healthandstability.com

Dr. Nick Bagnaro
Health and Stability Spinal Care
1650 N 32nd St
Muskogee, OK 74401
Phone: 918-991-5427
Fax: 877-335-6779
Email: drbagnaro@gmail.com
http://healthandstability.com

Dr. Nick Bagnaro
Health and Stability Spinal Care
232 S 7th St
Vinita, OK 74301
Phone: 918-991-5427
Fax: 877-335-6779
Email: drbagnaro@gmail.com
http://healthandstability.com

Dr. Raymond Marshall
Marshall Spinal Care
6931 S 66th East Avenue
Suite 200
Tulsa, OK 74133
Phone: 918 523-0111
Fax: 918 523-0312
Email: drraym@mac.com
http://www.marshallspinalcare.com

Dr. Rikki Sydebotham
Precision Spinal Health Care
1601 SE Washington Blvd.
Bartlesville, OK 74006
Phone: 918-331-9999
Fax: 918-331-9196
http://www.precisionspinalofbartlesville.com

Dr. T.C Sydebotham
Precision Spinal Health Care
1601 SE Washington Blvd.
Bartlesville, OK 74006
Phone: 918-331-9999
Fax: 918-331-9196
http://www.precisionspinalofbartlesville.com

Dr. Gregory Koors
Eugene Spinal Care
2201 Willamette St
Ste C
Eugene, OR 97405
Phone: 541-683-5678
Fax: 541-343-7350
Email: dockoors@yahoo.com
http://www.EugeneSpinalCare.com

Dr. Grant Dawson
Dawson Chiropractic Clinic
19767 SW 72nd Ave.
Suite 103
Tualatin, OR 97062
Phone: 503-620-6480
Fax: 503-684-4598
Email: dawsonchiropractic@gmail.com

Dr. Nicole Schmidt

Eugene Spinal Care
2201 Willamette St.
Suite C
Eugene, OR 97405
Phone: 541-683-5678
Fax: 541-343-7350
Email: nicoleschmidtdc@gmail.com
http://www.eugenespinalcare.com

Dr. Jordan Weeda
Wellspring Centre for Body Balance
108 E. Hersey St
Suite 2A
Ashland, OR 97520
Phone: 541.482.2021
Fax: 888.281.3789
Email: dr.jordan@wellspringbodybalance.com
http://www.wellspringbodybalance.com

Dr. Brad Hirschhorn
Hirschhorn Family Chiropractic Center
320 Huntingdon Pike
Rockledge, PA 19046
Phone: 215-663-8555
Fax: 215-663-8046
Email: bdhdc@verizon.net
Member Type: Gregory Circle Bronze Level JR
http://www.nuccadrbrad.com

Dr. David Gobbie

Balanced Health Chiropractic
850 Clairton Blvd
Ste 3200
Pittsburgh, PA 15236
Phone: 412-466-4930
Fax: 412-466-8274
Email: gobbiedc@hotmail.com
http://www.gobbiechiropractic.com

Dr. John Goodman
Chiropractic Head and Neck Treatment Center
427 W Main St
Ste. I
New Holland, PA 17557
Phone: 717-355-5575
Email: johngoody1982@yahoo.com
http://www.drjohngoodman.com

Dr. Timothy Strittmatter
Keystone Spinal Care
4000 Hempfield Plaza Boulevard, Suite 981
Greensburg, PA 15601
Phone: 724-216-9000
Fax: 724-216-9002
Email: keystonespinal@gmail.com
http://keystonespinal.com

Dr. Monika Franz
Franz Family Spinal Care
205 Bryce Circle
Suite A
Simpsonville, SC 29681
Phone: 864-987-5995
Fax: 864-987-5996
Email: drmonika@franzfamilyspinalcare.com
http://www.franzfamilyspinalcare.com

Dr. Benjamin Franz
Franz Family Spinal Care
205 Bryce Court
Suite A
Simpsonville, SC 29681
Phone: 864-987-5995
Fax: 864-987-5996
Email: drben@franzfamilyspinalcare.com
http://www.franzfamilyspinalcare.com

Dr. Jayson Snyder
Hartford Spinal Care
304 W. Hwy 38, Ste. 122
PO Box 446
Hartford, SD 57033
Phone: 605-528-6240
Fax: 605-528-6246
Email: lori@hartfordspinalcare.com
http://www.hartfordspinalcare.com
www.goodmanchiropracticmb.com

Dr. Shawn L Hall
Precision Spine Specialists
321 Billingsly Ct
Ste 14
Franklin, TN 37067
Phone: 615-778-0887
Fax: 615-778-0875
Email: drhall@precisionspineonline.com
http://www.precisionspineonline.com

Dr. Edward McCullough

McCullough Spinal Care
100 Commerce Drive
Suite B
Hendersonville, TN 37075
Phone: 615-264-8880
Fax: 615-264-8879
Email: doc@mcspinalcare.com
http://www.McSpinalCare.com

Dr. L. "Jake" McCullough
McCullough Spinal Care
100 Commerce Drive
Suite B
Hendersonville , TN 37075
Phone: 615-264-8880
Fax: 615-264-8879
Email: mcspinalcare@gmail.com
http://www.McSpinalCare.com

Dr. Patricia Gregg
1205 Nueces Street
Austin, TX 78701
Phone: 512-479-7878
Fax: 512-479-6280
Email: docnucca@bigplanet.com
http://backnbalance.biz

Dr. Janis Frahm
Back N Balance
1205 Nueces St.
Austin, TX 78701
Phone: 512-479-7878
Fax: 512-479-6280
Email: frahm_j@hotmail.com

Dr. Jason Minogue

Houston Spinal Care, PC
5715 Northwest Central Dr
Ste F-111
Houston, TX 77092
Phone: 713-690-4150
Fax: 713-690-4175
Email: drjason@hspinalcare.com
http://www.hspinalcare.com

Dr. Travis Rader
North Dallas Spine Center
7708 San Jacinto Place
Suite 300
Plano, TX 75024
Phone: 972-781-0010
Fax: 972-212-9378
Email: frontdesk@northdallasspinecenter.com
http://www.NorthDallasSpineCenter.com

Dr. D. Scott Sweeney
Back N' Balance
1205 Nueces Street
Austin, TX 78701
Phone: 512-479-7878
Fax: 512-479-6280
Email: dssweeney@sbcglobal.net

Dr. Cecilia Yu
Synergy Balance
12740 Hillcrest Road
Suite 138
Dallas, TX 75230
Phone: 972-387-4700
Fax: 972-387-4702
Email: C1@mysynergybalance.com

Dr. Jack Stockwell
Dr. Jack Stockwell & Associates
10714 South Jordan Gateway
Suite 220
Salt Lake City, UT 84095
Phone: 801-523-1890
Fax: 801-523-1495
Email: jack@jackstockwell.com
http://www.jackstockwell.com

Dr. Jack Stockwell
Dr. Jack Stockwell & Associates
188 North Bluff Street
St. George, UT 84770
Phone: (435) 688-1890
Email: sgoffice@jackstockwell.com
http://www.jackstockwell.com

Dr. Bryce Crowley
Davis County Spinal Care, P.C.
1134 West 500 North
Centerville, UT 84014
Phone: 801-294-6333
Fax: 801-294-8005
Email: drc@utahchiro.com
http://www.DCspinalcare.com

Dr. Craig Dawson
10714 S. Jordan Gateway
Ste. 220
South Jordan, UT 84095
Phone: 801-523-1890
Fax: 801-523-1495
Email: drcraigdawson@hotmail.com

Dr. Brent Noorda

Balanced Spinal Care
169 W 2710 South Cir
Ste. 204a
St. George, UT 84790
Phone: 435-688-2292
Fax: 435-688-2675
Email: Noorda@balancedspinalcare.com
http://balancedspinalcare.com

Dr. David Packer
Precision Spinal Care
1305 Executive Blvd.
Suite 170
Chesapeake, VA 23320
Phone: 757-382-5555
Fax: 757-382-5556
Email: nuccava@yahoo.com
http://www.nuccaspinalcare.com

Dr. Allen Harrison
Precision Spinal Care
1305 Executive Blvd.
Suite 170
Chesapeake, VA 23320
Phone: 757-382-5555
Fax: 757-382-5556
Email: dr.allenharrison@gmail.com
http://www.nuccaspinalcare.com

Dr. Michael Russamano

The Body Balancing Center
1410 Incarnation Drive
Suite 204
Charlottesville, VA 22901
Phone: 434-817-7788
Fax: 434-817-7750
Email: info@nuccavirginia.com
http://www.nuccavirginia.com

Dr. Jeremy Kerrigan
1305 Executive Blvd. Suite 170
Chesapeake, VA 23320
Phone: 757-382-5555
Fax: 757-382-5556
Email: jskerrigan@gmail.com
http://www.nuccaspinalcare.com

Dr. Vince Fitzpatrick
18211 E. Appleway Ave.
Spokane Valley, WA 99016
Phone: 509-926-1551
Fax: 509-926-1661
Email: drvfitz@comcast.net
http://www.nuccaspokanechiropractor.com

Dr. Johanna Hoeller
4345 Roosevelt Way NE
Seattle, WA 98105
Phone: 206-547-6370
Fax: 206-675-0890
Email: jhoellerdc@aol.com
http://www.NUCCAinSeattle.com

Dr. Craig Lapenski

Advanced Spinal Care
21806 - 103rd Ave. Ct. E.
Suite 101
Graham, WA 98338
Phone: 253-445-8181
Fax: 253-445-7938
Email: drlapenski@gmail.com
http://www.nuccawashington.com

Dr. Lee Yardley
Yardley Institute of UpperCervical Health Sciences
26238 Pacific Hwy South
Kent, WA 98032
Phone: 253-529-1100
Fax: 253-529-9825
Email: dryardley@me.com
http://www.yardleyinstitute.org

Dr. Margaret Burbidge
Complete Health Chiropractic
2004 E. Union Street
Seattle, WA 98122
Phone: 206-329-2892
Fax: 206-888-2343
Email: mburbidgedc@gmail.com
http://www.seattlecompletehealth.com

Dr. Robert Neff
Upper Cervical of Lynden, Inc.
115 7th Street
Lynden, WA 98264
Phone: 360-354-5341
Fax: 360-354-5341
Email: drneff@nucca.com
http://www.UCLynden.com

Dr. Justin Schallmann
Back In Balance Redmond Chiropractic
2761 152nd Ave NE
Redmond, WA 98052
Phone: 425-437-9974
Fax: 425-437-9964
Email: dcjustin@gmail.com
http://www.RedmondChiropractic.com

Dr. Kurt Sherwood
Sherwood Family Chiropractic PS
16810 - 108th Ave. S.E.
Renton, WA 98055
Phone: 425-227-0111
Fax: 425-228-2583
Email: drkurt@sherwoodchiropractic.com
http://www.sherwoodchiropractic.com

Dr. Chad Abramson
Abramson Family Chiropractic
10333 19th Ave. SE
Suite 103
Everett, WA 98208
Phone: 425-315-6262
Fax: 877-848-7680
Email: abramson@wwdb.org
http://www.nuccaclinic.com

Dr. Steven Glass

Glass Chiropractic Clinic
4407 N. Division St.
Suite 415
Spokane, WA 99207
Phone: 509-484-2044
Fax: 509-489-6733
Email: glasschiro@comcast.net
http://glasschiropractic.com

Dr. Traci Grandfield
Back In Balance
2761 152nd Avenue NE
Redmond , WA 98052
Phone: 425-437-9974
Fax: 425-437-9964
Email: grandfielddc@gmail.com
http://www.backinbalanceredmond.com

Dr. Derrick Hau
Vancouver Spinal Care
1610 C Street
Suite 103
Vancouver, WA 98663
Phone: 360-694-0300
Fax: 360-694-0301
Email: drhau@vancouverspinalcare.com
http://www.vancouverspinalcare.com

Dr. Lucas McCully
Yardley Institute of UpperCervical Health Sciences
26238 Pacific Hwy South
Kent, WA 98032
Phone: 253-529-1100
Email: mccullydc@gmail.com

Dr. Reanna Plancich

Discover Health Chiropractic PLLC
6739 15th Ave NW
Seattle, WA 98117
Phone: 206-577-3588
Fax: 206-577-3599
Email: drplancich@gmail.com
http://www.discoverhealthinseattle.com

Dr. Anni Ala
Complete Health Chiropractic
2004 East Union St.
Seattle, WA 98122
Phone: 206-329-2892
Email: annaladc@gmail.com
http://www.seattlecompletehealth.com

Dr. Earl Anderson
Anderson Health and Healing
323 Bambi Drive
Camano Island, WA 98282
Phone: 360-387-8124
Fax: 360-387-8124
Email: feelgreat@andersonhealthandhealing.com
http://www.andersonhealthandhealing.com

Dr. Sean Fryer
The Balanced Spine
22525 SE 64th Place
Suite 110
Issaquah, WA 98027
Phone: 425-369-1040
Fax: 425-369-1041
Email: info@thebalancedspine.com
http://www.TheBalancedSpine.com

Dr. Tim McFadden

InBalance Wellness Center
15600 Redmond Way
Suite 302
Redmond, WA 98052
Phone: 425-881-5811
Fax: 425-881-6220
Email: info@redmondspinalcare.com
http://www.RedmondSpinalCare.com

Dr. Julie Paul
Vancouver Spinal Care
1610 C. St. Suite 103
Vancouver, WA 98663
Phone: 360-694-0300
Fax: 360-694-0301
Email: drjuliepaul@gmail.com
http://www.vancouverspinalcare.com

Dr. Joseph Perin
Balanced Living Chiropractic
6405 NE 116 Ave
Ste 106
Vancouver, WA 98662
Phone: (360)597-4784
Email: drjoeperin@gmail.com
http://www.balancedlivingvancouver.com

Dr. Martha Schenk

Advanced Spinal Care
21806-103rd Ave Ct E
Ste #101
Graham, WA 98338
Phone: 253-445-8181
Fax: 253-445-7938
Email: dr.marthaschenk@gmail.com
http://www.nuccawashington.com

Dr. Steven Simmons
Valley Spinal Care
312 E. Trow Avenue
Suite 200
Chelan, WA 98816
Phone: (509) 888-9000
Fax: (509) 888-2412
Email: valleyspinalcare@hotmail.com
http://valleyspinalcare.net

Dr. Todd Smith
Bellingham Spinal Care
1633 Birchwood Ave.
Ste 102
Bellingham, WA 98225
Phone: 360-527-3668
Fax: 360-527-3668
Email: drtodd35@hotmail.com

Dr. Bryan R. Stewart
Stewart Family Chiropractic Clinic
547 Main Street
Edmonds, WA 98020
Phone: 425-672-4476
Email: bryan@nucca.net
http://WWW.Nucca.net

Dr. Chad Wheatley
Yardley Institute
26238 Pacific Hwy S
Kent, WA 98032
Email: drchadwheatly@gmail.com

Dr. Ryan Yates
Intelligent Balance Spinal Care & Wellness Center
2310 N Molter Rd
Suite 108
Liberty Lake, WA 99019
Phone: 509-924-4443
Fax: 509-924-1249
Email: dryates@spokanenucca.com

Dr. Lucas Watterson
Mountain State Wellness
965 Hartman Run Road
Suite 1101
Morgantown, WV 26505
Phone: 304-292-7740
Fax: 304-292-7741
Email: mtnstatewellness@aol.com
http://www.mtnstatewellness.com

Dr. Katherine Lord
Lord Spinal Care S.C.
5944 Seminole Centre Ct Suite 230
Fitchburg, WI 53711
Phone: 608-442-7400
Fax: 608-442-1105
Email: lordspinalcare@tds.net
http://www.lordspinalcare.com

Dr. Knut Feiker

Healing Point Chiropractic, LLC
10033 N. Port Washington Rd.
Mequon, WI 53092
Phone: 414-403-3612
Email: knutfeiker@gmail.com

Dr. Amber Pergande
Advanced Spinal Care, LLC
1052 Oak Forest Dr
Suite 210
Onalaska, WI 54650
Phone: 608 783-0384
Email: advancedspinalcare@yahoo.com

Dr. Travis Salisbury
Salisbury Clinic of Chiropractic
386 S. Koeller Street
Oshkosh, WI 54902
Phone: 920-651-0780
Fax: 920-651-0782
Email: tsalisburydc@yahoo.com

Dr. Dale Strama
Correction Creek Chiropractic Centre, LLC
1260 S. 8th St.
Medford, WI 54451
Phone: 715-748-6969
Fax: 715-748-3687
Email: ahwdale@tds.net

Dr. Clint Erickson, D.C., S.C.P.
Erickson Chiropractic
32 E 4th Ave
Afton, WY 83110
Phone: 307 885-9414
Email: svnuccadoc@gmail.com

APPENDIX B. NUCCA Practitioners U.K. and Canadian

Heidi Grant
NUCCA Chiropractor
Suite 21, Harcourt House
19 Cavendish Square
London W1G 0PL, UK
t +44 (0)20 7495 2206
e heidi@nucca.co.uk

(Heidi Grant is currently the only U.K. NUCCA Chiropractor)

Dr. Albert Berti
#103-6351 197th St
Langley, BC V2Y1X8
Phone: 604-533-0504
Fax: 604-533-0616
Email: BERTIAA@SHAW.CA

Dr. Richard De Camillis
101A - 3701 Hastings St.
Burnaby, BC V5C 2H6
Phone: 604-291-1166
Fax: 604-291-8182
Email: Drrick10@shaw.ca

Dr. D. Gordon Hasick

The Britannia Clinic
Suite 201- 5005 Elbow Dr., S.W.
Calgary, AB T2S 2T6
Phone: 403-243-0155
Fax: 403-243-0844
Email: info@c-1.com

Dr. Dan Erickson
Living Well Chiropractic
2010 Abbotsford Way
Abbotsford, BC V2S-6X8
Phone: 604-853-9898
Fax: 604-853-9801
Email: info@livingwellabbotsford.com

Dr. Michael Foran
8041 Granville St.
Vancouver, BC V6P 4Z5
Phone: 888-863-2537
Fax: 604-266-9622
Email: neckdr@shaw.ca
http://www.neckdr.com

Dr. Jeff Hedrich
Hedrich Chiropractic Acupuncture Shockwave
#204 740 4th Avenue South
Lethbridge, AB T1J 0N9
Phone: 403-381-2132
Fax: 403-524-4114
Email: drhedrich@shaw.ca
http://www.drhedrich.ca

Dr. Sloane Hunter

Align Health & Wellness
4 Parkdale Cres. NW
Calgary, AB T2N 3T8
Phone: (403) 452-4290
Fax: (403) 457-4299
Email: drsloanehunter@yahoo.ca
http://www.alignhealthandwellness.com

Dr. Blair Schmaus
Symmetry Spinal Care
7654-156 Street
Edmonton, AB T5R 4K7
Phone: 780-462-0447
Fax: 780-462-3219
Email: info@symmetryspinalcare.com
http://www.symmetryspinalcare.com

Dr. Shawn Thomas
Long Lake Chiropractic Centre
3955 Victoria Avenue
Nanaimo, BC V9T 2A1
Phone: 250-758-1531
Fax: 250-758-1532
Email: drsthomas@yahoo.com
http://www.myspine.ca

Dr. Gary Thomson
4835 woodridge court
Kelowna, BC V1W 3B4
Email: gnthom@shaw.ca

Dr. Travis Cox

Acadia Wellness Centre
#2, 430 Acadia Drive
Calgary, AB T2J 0B2
Email: drtwmcox@gmail.com
http://www.acadiawellness.com

Dr. Elaine Doyle
Unit 2- 373 Bridge Street West
Waterloo, ON N2K 3K3
Phone: 519-880-0260
Fax: 519-880-9615
Email: drdoyle@nucca.ca
http://www.nucca.ca

Dr. Janeen Hoffos
Acadia Wellness Centre
#2-430 Acadia Drive, S. E.
Calgary, AB T2J 0B2
Phone: 403-253-6785
Fax: 403-253-6280
Email: jhoffos@msn.com
http://www.acadiawellness.com

Dr. Franchesca Lee
Symmetry Spinal Care
7654 - 156 Street
Edmonton, AB T5R 4K7
Phone: 780-495-0028
Fax: 780-462-3219
Email: drfranchescalee@gmail.com
http://www.symmetryspinalcare.com

Dr. Brett Moore

275 Trafalgar Rd.
Oakville, ON L6J 3H1
Phone: 905-845-5747
Fax: 905-845-0306
Email: moorechiro@cogeco.net

Dr. Jim Moore
Moore Chiropractic Health Center
5912 Hazeldean Road
Ottawa, ON K2S 1B9
Phone: 613-831-8374
Fax: 613-831-0812
Email: jandcmoore@rogers.com

Dr. Jeffrey Scholten
Practice of Upper Cervical Chiropractic
Northland Professional Building - Suite 104
4600 Crowchild Trail NW
Calgary, AB T3A 2L6
Phone: 403-247-4257
Fax: 403-247-4275
Email: info@drscholten.com
http://www.drscholten.com

Dr. Tania Siqueira
Life Balance Chiropractic & Wellness Centre
1370 Don Mills Rd.
Ste. 205
North York, ON M3B 3N7
Phone: 416-445-9355
Fax: 416-445-3300
Email: tani_siqueira@yahoo.com
http://www.nuccatoronto.com

Dr. Jean-Paul Bohemier

Practice of Upper Cervical Chiropractic
Northland Professional Building
Suite 104-4600 Crowchild Trail NW
Calgary, AB T3A 2L6
Phone: 403-247-4257
Fax: 403-247-4275
Email: nucca.dr.bohemier@gmail.com
http://www.drbohemier.com

Dr. Dustin Freund
Living Well Clinic
2010 Abbotsford Way
Abbotsford, BC V2F 6X8
Phone: 604-853-9898
Email: info@livingwellabbotsford,com
http://www.livingwellabbotsford.com

Dr. Christiane Gendron
Kirospecifik Sherbrooke
2244 King West Street
Sherbrooke, QC J1J2E8
Phone: 819 820 2242
Email: kiro.cg@gmail.com
http://www.kirosherbrooke.com

Dr. Clint Hallgrimson
Functional Upper Cervical Chiropractic
#104 1635 Abbott St.
Kelowna, BC V1Y 1A9
Phone: 250-763-1152
Fax: 250-763-1187
Email: dr.clint@shaw.ca

Dr. Mylene Hopf

Practice of Upper Cervical Chiropractic
Northland Professional Building
Suite 104, 4600 Crowchild Trail NW
Calgary, AB T3A 2L6
Phone: 403-247-4257
Fax: 403-247-4275
Email: mylenehopf@gmail.com
http://www.drhopf.com

Dr. Philip Kanwischer
2336 156th Street
Surrey, BC V4A 4V4
Phone: 604-536-6333
Email: philk@telus.net

Dr. Bradley Kennedy
PrecisionSpinalCare
#101 - 51 Sunpark Drive SE
Calgary, AB T2X 3V4
Phone: 403-201-1954
Fax: 888-201-1724
Email: chirobradley@gmail.com
http://www.drbradleykennedy.ca

Dr. Benjamin Kuhn
Providence Chiropractic Clinic
4556 - 99 Street
Edmonton, AB T6E 5H5
Phone: 780-450-1041
Fax: 780-450-2156
Email: dr.kuhn@providencenucca.com
http://www.providencenucca.com

Dr. Randy Mills

Dr. Randy Mills Chiropractic Inc.
443 Carney St.
Prince George, BC V2M 2K4
Phone: 250-563-4563
Fax: 250-563-1603
Email: drmills@telus.net

Dr. Russill Mills
443 Carney St
Prince George, BC V2M2K4
Phone: 250-563-4563
Fax: 250-563-4563
Email: russillmills@gmail.com

Dr. Aurora Ongaro
Symmetry Spinal Care
7654 156th St
Edmonton, AB T5R4K7
Phone: 780-442-0030
Email: auroraongaro@hotmail.com
http://www.symmetryspinalcare.com

Dr. Mikael Reney
Centre Kiro Spécifik
1755 boul. du Souvenir
Laval, QC H7N 5V5
Phone: 450-668-8777
Email: mr@kiro.ca
http://www.kiro.ca

Dr. Ankur Tayal

UC Life Chiropractic Centre
1-1113 Langley Street
Victoria, BC V8W 1V9
Phone: 250-386-5433
Email: drtayal@uclife.ca
http://www.uclife.ca

Dr. Jamie Thomson
10A-1380 Summit Drive
Kamloops, BC V2C 1T8
Phone: 250-374-3522
Fax: 250-372-8098
Email: thomson-nicholson@shaw.ca

APPENDIX C. Typical Causes of Upper Cervical Displacement

Atlas displacement can be caused by a variety of circumstances. Adding to the puzzle is that injury will often occur years before symptoms manifest themselves. The insidious condition slowly worsens over time and the patient often does not realize what is happening until it becomes a serious condition. Patients will often have one of these incidents in their past often years or decades before the condition degenerates to the point of seeking medical help.

Trauma to the head at birth
Involvement in a motor vehicle accident
A fall
A blow to the head
An unusual twist of the body often with a "cracking noise"
Frontal whiplash from any cause
Lateral whiplash from any cause
Injury caused by an uneven surface
Occupation with repetitive motions
Sedentary Occupation

APPENDIX D. Typical Symptoms of Upper Cervical Displacement

The condition can present itself in a variety of ways. It is not unusual to experience multiple symptoms in combination. Here are a few of the many possibilities.

Headaches from unknown cause
Migraine headaches from unknown cause
Neck pain
Shoulder pain
Fatigue
Drooping shoulder
Constant pain from "everywhere"
Random shooting pain in extremities
Racing heart from minimal exertion
Foggy vision
Brain "fog"
Flashes of light in vision
Eyes adjust slowly to light
Ringing in the ears
Staggered gait
Difficulty with balance
Dizziness
Incontinence
Numbness and tingling sensations
One leg apparently shorter than the other
Sensation of pin pricks on bottom of feet
Pain in the hips
Panic Attacks
Difficulty concentrating
Slow thought process
Intolerance to heat and cold
Intolerance to light

Intolerance to sound
Shaking hands
Muscle spasms
Jaw misalignment
Tooth pain
Discolored hands
Short term memory loss
Stomach Pain
"Knot" in stomach
Slow reflexes
Difficulty standing for prolonged period of time
Scratchy throat
Raspy voice
Pain in head when lying down

APPENDIX E. Typical Symptoms During Recovery

Recovery from atlas displace can be just as bizarre as the original symptoms. Here are some of the things that may happen to you.

Feeling of pin pricks on skin
Sensation of flashes of heat on skin
Difficulty with balance
Flashes of light in vision
Shooting pain alternating from left to right extremities
Difficulty adjusting to temperature changes
Muscle cramps
Pain that comes and goes
Lack of endurance
Change in sense of taste and smell

APPENDIX F. Activities Which Can Activate Symptoms

A wide variety of motions can cause difficulty with an atlas displacement condition. These are also good indicators of the condition. Avoiding these activities during recovery can help control the pain.

Lifting
Driving
Sitting for a prolonged period
Lying down
Turning the head
Holding the head still (such as in a theatre)
Walking on an uneven surface
Walking up steps
Leaning forward

ABOUT THE AUTHOR

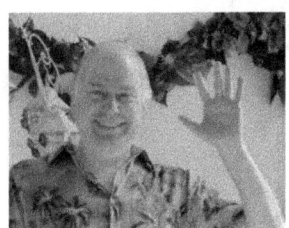

Edmund S. Figure is a graduate of the University of Michigan with a degree in Business Administration and a major in Finance. He worked for over 30 years in the technical side of the financial industry before retiring at a young age to become a self-employed entrepreneur.

In his financial works *The Dividend Gold Mine, The Dividend Gold Mine II,* and *The Dividend Gold Mine III* he describes for the new and experienced investor a time proven method of accumulating a lifetime of wealth in the stock market using the immense power of compounded dividends.

In the *Dividend Gold Mine* series in plain simple language you'll learn how to avoid market pitfalls and how to recover from them. Also included are the only option strategies you'll ever need to profit further from your dividend portfolio. He draws on his investing experience to share a lifetime of lessons learned so that you can avoid market pitfalls on your way to creating your own wealth using a steady stream of dividend income.

His previous works includes *How I Overcame Fibromyalgia* in which he describes overcoming the obstacles he found in the health care establishment and "A Psychic Adventure" which is the culmination of a lifetime of observing paranormal events.

He also shares his experiences with young readers in *The Baseball Kid* in his *Lifelong Lessons* series. In *The Baseball Kid* young readers live the highs and lows of trying to become a professional baseball player.